THE STRENGTH WITHIN: OVERCOMING BREAST CANCER

A PERSONAL DIARY

LESLIE WILSON

ISBN eBook: 979-8-218-58765-9
ISBN Paperback: 979-8-218-58622-5
ISBN Hardcover: 979-8-9923556-8-0

CONTENTS

DEDICATION

To the warriors who face a breast cancer diagnosis with courage and resilience, this book is for you. Your strength is a testament to the indomitable human spirit. May you find hope, comfort, and inspiration within these pages as you navigate your journey.

To the caregivers, family members, and friends who stand by their loved ones through every step of the battle, your unwavering support and love are the pillars that uphold those in need. Your compassion and dedication are invaluable, and this book is a tribute to your selfless acts of kindness.

Together, we are stronger. Together, we fight. Together, we live..
.

PREFACE

In the middle of the night, I was jolted awake by a vivid dream. Grabbing the journal pad from my nightstand, I scribbled down the words "Chosen One." In my dream, I was enveloped in darkness, and a voice echoed clearly, "Chosen One." When morning came, I realized that this was not just a title for the book everyone had been urging me to write—it was a divine message. God was telling me that I was chosen for a purpose far greater than I could have imagined.

If you're reading this book, you might be facing a breast cancer diagnosis, supporting a loved one through their battle, or simply seeking to understand this journey. You may be feeling a whirlwind of emotions—fear, anger, confusion, or even defiance. How did this happen to you? Why were you dealt this hand? How will you navigate this life-altering path? And most importantly, will you choose to fight like hell to LIVE?

I chose to fight. This book is a raw, unfiltered account of my journey through breast cancer. It began as a way to keep my family informed without having to repeat my story endlessly. But it quickly evolved into something much more profound. As the "Chosen One," I was called to share my truth, to be transparent and visible, and to give a voice to those who struggle to find the words.

Through daily blog entries, I documented my thoughts, interactions, medical decisions, treatments, and side effects. This is not your typical cancer story. It's an honest, heartfelt blueprint for patients and caregivers alike, offering a glimpse into the reality of living with breast cancer. Join me on this journey, and together, we will find the strength to fight and the courage to live.

INTRODUCTION

I'm a Survivor

It's January 2010 and I have decided that I will lose 20lbs by the end of March. That's right I want to return to high school skinny. My days over the next couple of months is consumed with counting calories and exercising to reach my ideal body weight.

Fast-forward, now it's the beginning of March and I have reached my weight loss goal ahead of schedule. Spring always seems to energize me, so I begin a series of vacations. There is a spontaneous trip home to help Dad celebrate his 35th job anniversary, a birthday cookout at my home for my friends, an Aries Birthday Bash in New Orleans, and then off to explore DC and Virginia with my extended family. Yes, Spring is definitely in the air and I'm planning to enjoy every moment of it. I feel like I'm on top of the world. It's Memorial Day and I eagerly rush off to Aruba for my annual girl's trip. As always, the time goes by too fast and before I know it I'm back to work and being Mommy. Yet, I begin planning my next adventure. I schedule what I call "Leslie's Road trip" and invite friends from Virginia, Washington, DC, & North Carolina to join me in Charleston, SC for a Father's Day Bash.

I complete another exhausting work week, take a shower, jump in bed and perform my monthly breast self-exam. What is this? I feel something in my right breast but not sure what it is. It almost feels like a pulled muscle. Hmm that's odd but I'm sure it is a pulled muscle or something. Since I'm no breast expert and have no clue about what I think I might be feeling, I'll call my gynecologist in the morning just to be sure. Surprisingly, the next day I'm able to get an afternoon appointment. My doctor is not concerned about what she feels but agrees to send me to an imaging center. By the end of the week, I have a mammogram and ultrasound. The doctor informs me that they are pretty sure I have breast cancer, but a biopsy will be required to confirm. What???!!!??? This can't be real. I exercise. I don't smoke. I cook healthy meals full of organic fruits and vegetables. I'm the family health nut that everyone makes fun of. This cannot be real. I allow myself to cry for about 20 minutes as I decide how to break this news to my family. The tears are not for my own sorrow but for the pain this will cause to all of those who love me. I'm always the one that protects and nurtures everyone and I know this is something that I cannot protect them from. I decided to make a conference call between my parents and sisters to share the news with everyone at the same time. I allow them to spend the night crying and dealing with the shock before I arrive the next day for the Father's Day Road trip as planned.

I've always been an optimistic person and don't worry about things that I have no control over. We enjoyed a weekend with family and friends full of laughter, food, dancing, and drinks. After the bash, I return home for my biopsy. Now, it's my parents' wedding anniversary and I must call them with the news, I have been diagnosed with breast cancer. Now, I break the news to my children and then my friends. After the initial shock, there are many emotions that overwhelm me. I'm angry, I'm mad as hell, I'm scared, and I'm worried. I begin to wonder, what was the point for me trying to live a wholesome life to be repaid in this manner. Then as quickly as these thoughts come to me, I push them aside and move into fight mode. Yes, bad things do happen to good people. Maybe my healthy lifestyle was instrumental in preventing the disease from spreading and it will allow me to heal quickly. God is still in charge. I plan a pre-chemo dinner party and go to the barber and shave my hair off. I'm ready to win this fight and I refuse to be down or allow anyone to have a pity party.

Now that I reflect on my life in the months before diagnosis, the advice that I would give to myself is to keep on doing what you are doing. Remain focused on preventative health exams, exercising, and eating properly. Continue your passion for enjoying the present and living a full life. Do not allow negative people, negative situations, or any negative energy to occupy any space in your life. Be open to letting new friends in and letting go of others. But most importantly Live Now! Do not wait for your kids to finish school, Live Now! Do not wait until you reach that milestone birthday, Live Now! Do not wait until you are married,
Live Now!
Live Now!
Live Now!
Live Now!

1 THE DIAGNOSIS

Discover Lump 6/14/2010

While going to bed, I discover what I believe to be a lump in my right breast. I'm not really sure because I'm far from a breast expert but I sent myself an email to my work address to remind myself to make an appointment with my doctor to check it out. When in doubt seek advice from the experts. If you want to know about crack, then you go to a crack head. If you want to know about breast, then you go to the breast doctor. - Leslie
  Michelle

GYN Exam - 6/15/2010

I called my Gyn to request an exam because I might have discovered a lump. Today, must be my "lucky" day because there was a cancellation on her books, and she could see me at 12:15pm. During the visit, she was not concerned about the lump but as a precaution scheduled an appointment for me at an Imaging Clinic for a mammogram & ultrasound. It is highly unlikely that my doctor would have discovered this during my annual visit. It took me awhile to relocate it again.

'If you don't know your body don't expect anyone else to". ~Leslie Michelle

Mammogram/Ultrasound - 6/17/2010

Went to the Paredes Imaging Clinic for Women to have a mammogram & ultrasound. I was in for the shock of my life. The doctor met with me at the end of the examination and informed me that there was a 80 - 90% chance that the lump I discovered was cancer due to the jagged edges of the tumor. She scheduled a biopsy for the following week to determine if in fact the tumor is cancerous or not. The hardest part of this day was calling my family to break the news to them. I scheduled a conference call with my Mom & sisters. parents, sisters, & brother-in-law. I decided that I would not tell my children until after the results of the biopsy. My emotions/thoughts - this can't be real. I'm the health nut in the family. Should I tell anyone or keep it to myself? What to expect from others - complete shock, speechlessness, & tears. I can still hear my Mom gasping for air while trying to remain calm for my benefit.

Biopsy - 6/23/2010

My cousin, Moni came to town to be with me during my ultrasound-guided biopsy. I was incredibly nervous. Most women I think would have the fear of someone sticking a needle in such a sensitive area. For the men, reviewing this entry I imagine it would be the same fear if you knew someone was sticking a needle in your testicles. The biopsy was not bad at all. The first needle was local anesthesia to numb the area which was followed by another needle to withdraw tissue. All of this was done while the nurse was guiding the doctor to the location by using an ultrasound. What did it feel like? Anesthesia is like

1

getting Novocain at the dentist office & you don't feel the biopsy at all. The entire process took about 30 minutes. After the biopsy I had to sit for another 30 minutes with an ice pack which was followed by a mammogram. At the biopsy, I learned that a steel marker was left inside my body so that it would be easier for doctors to zone in on this location during future exams.

~ Wonder if this is a government conspiracy to place a GPS in my body. Only kidding - got to have a little humor ~Leslie Michelle

Biopsy Results - 6/24/2010
Today is my parents' anniversary as well as the day that I received confirmation that I do indeed have Stage I - Breast Cancer. I dreaded making the call to let my family know the news. What was my reaction? Shock, overwhelmed with questions and random thoughts. What did I do? I cried for about 20 minutes and then went to the bar for 4 shots of Grey Goose with Moni & Ana. Now the pity party is over, I refuse to let ANYTHING steal my joy.

"My focus is on living a full life and not the hurdles that I cross along the way". ~ Leslie Michelle

Informing my Children 6/25/2010
I have four teenagers. Two biological daughters & an adopted daughter and son that I have been raising since their mother's death in 2005. Their ages are 17, 14, 12, & 12. I sat my children down for a family meeting with my mom, one of my sister's, and my nephews and told them this: "I discovered a small lump in my breast, it has cancer cells present, I'm going to be okay but will have surgery to remove the tumor. I will be tired and need your help while I'm healing". To my surprise the girls handled the news better than the adults. They are a very strong bunch and are eager to help me heal. My son, who is adopted, took the news very hard. He has already lost one mother and the fear of losing another mother is on his mind.

MRI - 6/28/2010

My doctor gave me anxiety pills to take before the MRI since I am like most folks, claustrophobic. An IV was inserted into my arm and then I entered the machine. It had more room than I expected. You are lying on a table stomach down with your boobies falling through two openings. Ear plugs are placed in your ears because of the loud popping noise while in the machine. The first 14 minutes passed then a substance referred to as contrast was run through my IV. This is to allow better images when taking the remainder of the pictures. The entire process takes approximately 30 minutes, and you are in absolutely no pain or discomfort. The most difficult part of this test is lying still with the annoying noise which sounds like pots and pans beating around your head. The technician called me approximately 30 minutes after I left the office because she was too excited to wait any longer. Good News - the tumor is local and has not spread to any parts of my body and does not appear to be in any lymph nodes.

Surgeon Consultation - 6/30/2010

The imaging clinic provided me with a follow-up appointment with a surgeon, but I reached out to my family & friends for references in my city as well. A friend, who works in breast cancer research, suggested Dr. Polly Stephens at St. Francis. My Mom and one of my sisters joined me for the consultation.

Prior to arriving, I assumed that I would elect to have a mastectomy. I felt that this was the best option for all breast cancer patients. After meeting with the surgeon and staff, I was persuaded that I did not need to have such a radical procedure after all. My cancer is small, was caught early, and has not spread to any lymph nodes. It is recommended that I have a lumpectomy with radiation and possibly chemo. I agree with this recommendation and schedule my surgery for July 8th. I also took the screening test for BRAC I & II which is a genetic mutation known to be linked to breast cancer. This test is important to me because I have two younger sisters as well as two biological daughters. The results should arrive within two weeks.

"Be cautious regarding who you accept advice from. Many will offer their opinions, but a very few are even qualified". ~ Leslie Michelle

"Every case and circumstance is different. Do what is best for you & in your situation." Leslie Michelle

Self-Exam - 7/4/2010

Reminder: Self-Exams are IMPORTANT. I believe it is even more important than your annual pap smear yet so few people perform them. I'm not old enough to have an annual mammogram but I have breast cancer. I go to all of my doctor appointments but none of them discovered my lump. Teach your daughters, sisters, nieces, mothers, grandmothers, cousins, friends, fathers, brothers, nephews, uncles, and grandfathers to perform self-exams once a month. Breast cancer can occur at any age and to anybody. Early detection starts with you!

"Your body is your body. Know your body, look at your body, touch your body, and if there is any doubt about what you discover go to the doctor and have a professional check it out". ~ Leslie Michelle

Aches after Biopsy - 7/5/2010

It has been 12 days since I had my biopsy and I'm still feeling the effects. The pain or ache is random and occurs if I try to lift anything over about 15lbs. I've also noticed that the aches occur when the AC is blowing directly on me in the car. This is frustrating the HELL out of me because my activities are limited.

Insurance - 7/6/2010

Forms, forms, forms and more forms. I'm thankful that I have a job and benefits but WOW trying to maneuver through the process is insane. Contact your boss, contact HR, complete the online form via Aetna's website for FMLA & short-term disability. Today, I discovered that Aetna's online form may provide a benefit for someone but not the sick because it simply initiates manual forms which arrived today. I got everything completed and faxed to my doctor and insurance company.

2 LUMPECTOMY

Preparing for surgery - 7/6/2010

I spent the day trying to get everything in order as I prepared for my surgery which is only 2 days away now. I had my doctor call in a prescription for pain meds so I can pick it up the day before my surgery. I'm trying to make sure that I have as many things completed in advance so that I'm not having to rely on other people for my errands. I spoke to a family member and another friend today and both confessed that they do not perform self-exams. Another friend called to pray with me over the phone and I was truly blessed. Many of you have indicated that you are not doing self-exams because you are not sure what to do. How about this; at your next gynecologist visit volunteer to demonstrate your self-exam technique with your doctor so he/ she can provide you with constructive feedback. Mystery solved - take charge! ~ Leslie Michelle

Pathology Details - 7/7/2010

I just received a call from my doctor regarding my surgery tomorrow. The details from my pathology report indicate that my tumor is estrogen/progesterone negative & HER2 positive. My type of cancer is called invasive ductal carcinoma. So what does all of this mean? During surgery tomorrow, I will have a lumpectomy (remove the tumor and surrounding tissue), a sentinel lymph node biopsy (the first lymph node that drains the breast is identified and removed), & a Port-a-Cath installed which will make it easier for me to receive chemo. Yes, chemotherapy will begin approximately 3 weeks after my surgery. Typically, symptoms experienced are loss of energy & loss of hair.

Headed to the hospital 7/8/2010

Last night I had so much fun being silly with my mom, sisters, and daughters. My son is at an AAU Basketball tournament in Myrtle Beach and has been calling to check on me daily. My Dad, brother-in-law, and nephews remained in Charleston but are with me in spirit. Today is the day that I have my lumpectomy. I'm feeling a little anxious because I don't know what to expect regarding the Port-a-Cath which will be installed. I must be at the hospital at 8 am & surgery begins at 10 am. It is expected to last for 2hrs. Thanks so much for all of the blog comments, prayers, emails, calls, and sharing the word about the importance of self-exams. I can't wait to tell you all about the surgery later today.
Love You All

How am I supposed to be cute or smell good during my surgery when they do not allow lotion, deodorant, nail polish, and perfume? It is killing me not to put some coconut oil on my skin.

Back Home 7/8/2010

I've just arrived home from my surgery. God is Good! The surgery confirmed my staging which is Stage I and the lymph node did not contain any cancer cells. Sandie the volunteer working in outpatient registration was also amazing. She had a wealth of information and is a survivor who was originally diagnosed with breast cancer at age 17. After the surgery, I woke up to pain but received some meds via the IV and took my pain pills. The port in my chest as well as the incision point in my neck is slightly uncomfortable but not painful. My doctor and the entire hospital staff were amazing! My meds are kicking in now so I will talk to you later.

My First Night 7/9/2010

I've been taking it easy, and I know that it is hard for everyone to believe. Blame it on the anesthesia and hydrocodone. I have not been nauseous, which is a blessing. Chicken noodle soup, crackers, ginger ale, & a slice of my sour cream pound cake. (Yes, I baked it before the surgery and didn't tell anyone). I have three incisions. 1) Right breast - lumpectomy - where the lump was removed and a lymph node for testing 2) left side of my chest where the port was installed 3) left area below collarbone where Port-a-Cath was installed through my jugular vein. Most of the discomfort I'm experiencing is in my neck from the incision in my jugular vein. It bothers me the most when I chew or turn my neck. Tomorrow, I will try not to take any prescription drugs and move to the over-the-counter meds. My mom, sisters, and daughters are taking wonderful care of me which is not easy. You all know I'm a control freak and they are quite upset that the drugs are not impacting my memory. Oh yeah, I forgot to tell you during the surgery they ran blue dye through my IV. This allowed my lymph nodes to be highlighted and show if there was any cancer present. God is Good - all lymph nodes were cancer-free. But guess what the side effects of the dye are? That's right, my urine is BLUE. I'm talking about turquoise/ultra blue. Of course, my inquisitive sister, Shana wanted to accompany me to the bathroom so she could see. LOL - I told you I would keep it REAL and give you all the details. Goodnight

Checking out my incisions 7/9/2010

I started my day by taking a shower and removing all of the adhesives that remained from the IV and heart monitor. The incisions were stitched internally and will dissolve. Externally, there was surgical glue used to close the incision points. The glue will eventually fall off as well. While taking my shower, I accidentally hit the port. Did you hear me scream? I'm sure I will not make that same mistake again! My neck is incredibly sore, and it is difficult to turn and bend. My throat is sore as well - I'm assuming from tubes that were inserted during the operation. I was stunned to see that my breast still looks the same as it did before the surgery. I thought a large indention would appear as though I was bitten by a shark or something. Nope - the only evidence is the incision, but my boobies are intact. I made my mom & sisters come take a look when I stepped out of the shower. Of course, my mom doesn't want me to put all of these details on the site but I told her there was a disclaimer on my welcome page. Besides, I want to make sure you have all of the details that may often be left out of other sites. How am I feeling? I'm a little nauseated today & sore. My neck gets tired if I'm up too long and I have to lay down. Guess my big head is weighing down on the incision. I'm trying to endure the pain without medication but I'm not sure how far I will make it. No meds & no Grey Goose - what will I do?

Rough Morning 7/10/2010
I woke up at 5:45 am due to excessive pain. I had to take my meds because everything was hurting. I find that it is more comfortable if I sleep with a bra on. My guess is that the support eliminates pressure on the incision. I've always felt that looking good helps to lift your spirits when you are not feeling well. So, I ate breakfast, took a shower, and got dressed including my dangles. Mind over matter!

Thankful for Family & Friends 7/11/2010
I'm so THANKFUL for my family & friends. I'm talking about the REAL people in our lives who just show up and do. Helping me with meals, my laundry, making sure I have my favorite foods, volunteering to get me to doctor appointments, and all of the laughter. Although some of you are taking advantage of the fact that I cannot defend myself right now. You know I'm a control freak so it's not funny for you to rearrange things in my house just for the HELL of it. LOL

~True friends are a rare jewel. I'm so glad that I discovered you!~
   Leslie Michelle

~My Family are those who come when I tell them don't. They
   do when I tell them don't. They give unconditionally and
   unselfishly and expect nothing in return. ~ Leslie Michelle

Sister Love 7/11/2010
While my sisters were in town for my surgery, they decided to dye a couple of their dreads pink to show their support. I can imagine the stares they will get from strangers and their co-workers. That is true love walking around looking like punk rockers from the 80s! LOL - Love You Sissy#1 & Sissy #2.

Thanks Joel Osteen 7/12/2010
I was a little depressed yesterday. I took a nap and dreamed that I was back to my normal active self. When I awoke to feel the port sticking out of my chest,

it was a slap of reality that I was not prepared for. Yet, God always shows up on time. I turned on my tv and one of my favorite ministers to watch, Joel Osteen came on. His message spoke directly to me. Programming Your Mind for Victory - Focus on the positive and not the negative. Believe that you are healed, and you are healed. Our God controls it all. We are victors and not victims. Remain in your place of peace and refuse to be frustrated, angry, or upset. When your mind focuses on positive thoughts, it sends signals to the rest of your body to act accordingly.

~I expect to be strong, healed, and full of energy. My mind will remain focused and connected to the promises of God. ~ Leslie Michelle

How to examine your breasts 7/12/2010
Performing regular breast self-exams can help you detect changes early. Look at your breasts for any changes in size, shape, contour, dimpling, redness, or scaliness of the nipple or breast skin.

Here's a step-by-step guide:

In the Shower: Use the pads of your three middle fingers to check the entire breast and armpit area. Apply light, medium, and firm pressure in a vertical pattern (up and down). Feel for any lumps, thickening, or hardened knots.

In Front of a Mirror: Visually inspect your breasts with your arms at your sides. Look for any changes in contour, swelling, dimpling, or skin changes. Next, raise your arms slightly overhead and look for the same changes. Finally, rest your palms on your hips and press firmly to flex your chest muscles, looking for any changes in the shape or contour of your breasts.

Lying Down: When lying down, the breast tissue is spread out evenly along the chest wall. Place a pillow under your right shoulder and your right arm behind your head. Using your left hand, move the pads of your fingers around your right breast gently in small circular motions covering the entire breast and armpit area. Use light, medium, and firm pressure. Squeeze the nipple to check for discharge and lumps. Repeat these steps on each breast.

Great News - BRAC negative 7/12/2010
The doctor just called to tell me that my genetic testing for BRAC I & II is negative. This is the gene mutation that is hereditary and typically indicates that you have a 100% chance of getting the disease in your breast or ovaries. This is wonderful news for my daughters, sisters, and me!

Full Pathology Report 7/13/2010

The full pathology report from surgery is just in. The results are good. My actual tumor size was 3.2cm which makes me a Stage II. What is more important is that the lymph nodes are all clear - no cancer was found. The test also showed that there is no need for additional surgery. The doctor is trying to get me into a targeted 5-day radiation therapy program. I hope to meet with the radiologist this week or next week.

Preparing for therapy 7/14/2010

I've spent most of the morning handling administrative affairs. Calls to Aetna to understand why my request for Short Term Disability / FMLA is still in a pending status. Yes, this is extremely frustrating and there should be an easier way to handle the paperwork BUT I'm thankful that I have insurance when so many do not. Moved my dental checkup so I can have my cleaning done before beginning chemo. Coordinating the timing of my appointments with the radiologist, oncologist, and surgeon. I will meet with the radiologist on Tuesday, July 20th. Dr. Douglas Arthur is top in the nation and will decide if I can have the 5-day targeted radiation therapy. If I'm approved for the targeted radiation therapy then I will have to return to my surgeon to have my incision reopened and a balloon inserted. This is a time-sensitive decision and has to be done within 3 weeks of the lumpectomy. Of course, I will provide you with all of the details regarding the radiation treatment after a decision is made on which therapy I will receive. No need to bore you with all the details too soon.

What does it feel like? 7/14/2010

I will try to include entries regarding questions I receive but some are often afraid to ask or to discuss. I will continue to work hard not to leave any stone unturned. One question, I have received on several occasions is "How did you feel, were there any symptoms?"

Before Diagnosis
I was the picture of good health. Healthy eating, don't let things stress me out, exercise, no sodas, limited sugar intake. Natural shampoos, lotions, deodorants. You name it, I did it.

After Biopsy
The breast will be sore. Random aches. May have to wait a few days to drive - I never realized how much your arm rubs against your breast during normal movements.

After Lumpectomy
My breast feels like a water balloon because fluid builds. I've been living in a bra because you appreciate the extra support in carrying the extra wait plus it

eliminates extra pressure against the incision. Yuck - I hate bras but now they are my "bestest" friend. Under my arm is sore due to the Sentinel Lymph Node Biopsy. My neck gets tired almost a cramping feeling. It feels better for me to sit where I can lay my head back against something like a pillow. The port in my chest feels like something creepy crawly is underneath my skin. So if you should happen to see me showing some weird behaviors like holding my boobie or turning my whole body rather than just my neck now you will understand why. I'm not completely psycho just trying to get comfortable in my new gear. LOL

Feeling Blessed 7/15/2010

In all things, I will continue to give him praise! Last night, I watched the movie, Living Proof starring Harry Connick, Jr . It was about the making of Herceptin which is the targeted therapy given to patients who are HER2 positive, like me. Wow - This gave me a new list of items to be thankful for.

Today I'm thankful for:
1. Testing for HER2 became a standard in 1998; without knowing what type of breast cancer you have, it is impossible to receive proper treatment.
2. Herceptin - the drug developed to fight HER2 positive breast cancer.
3. Dr. Dennis Slamon, the doctor who fought to have Herceptin approved by the FDA in 1998.
4. .Those women before me who agreed to be apart of the initial trial.
5. That I was chosen to carry this burden and not my daughters, sisters, mothers, or friends.

Aetna Hell 7/16/2010

I've spent the last day and a half dealing with Aetna. They need tons of forms, dates of doctor appointments, etc. They don't seem to understand why I could not come to work in between procedures. INSANITY!!! It is stuff like this that will make a person go postal. I've been told that I will have to get new forms and out-of-office dates for each of my treatments, radiation & chemo.

~ Maybe I should write a letter to my President and ask him to update the Health Care Reform bill to ensure that common sense practices are included in determination of short term disability. ~Leslie Michelle

My First Drive 7/17/2010

Today was my first time driving since the surgery. I think I did pretty well. LOL - I had to make minor adjustments like placing the seatbelt under my arm rather than across my chest. I can't take the pressure against the port. My neck is still not right yet so I'm limited with checking over my shoulder. So when you are praying for me again - make sure you ask Jesus to watch over me on the road. Where did I go? To a Hibachi restaurant for sushi & to the grocery store for some fruit. It felt good to be out of the house for a little while.

Still Being Me 7/18/2010

Wondering why I'm smiling and laughing? During my initial consultation with my surgeon, she was astonished to come into the room and hear me laughing with my mom & sister. You see, I'm sure it was not the norm in the VA Breast Center. But, I refuse to walk around feeling sorry for myself. Do I have moments of frustration? Absolutely, but I only allow them to occur for a moment. I refuse to stay in an atmosphere of negative energy. Through Jesus Christ, I am prepared for whatever comes my way. As illustrated in the bible, there are serpents that often come into our lives, right before God is about to show up with a blessing. My serpent right now is breast cancer. I'm claiming Victory through my faith and I will remain focused on my goals and not the hurdles that come along the way. I will continue to be "ME". I refuse to be molded by breast cancer into a person that I am not! Today I'm inspired by my cousin, Olivia McClurkin who was diagnosed with Stage IV breast cancer and given a few months to live. Olivia lived for 9 years astonishing all of her doctors. She has left a beautiful song as a symbol of her journey, The Healing Song. Have a blessed day!

Eating before chemo 7/19/2010

Today my cravings have been insane & I have given in to all of them. For lunch I was craving olive oil & bread from a local Italian restaurant. For dinner, fried chicken with fresh pineapples, crunchy Cheetos topped with Worcestershire sauce, and birthday cake. I know it is INSANE but that's what I wanted today! I'll probably be sick as a dog before tonight is over.

Food for Thought: There is scientific evidence that suggests that extra virgin olive oil kills HER2 breast cancer cells, so I'm going to listen to the desires of my stomach today. https://pubmed.ncbi.nlm.nih.gov/19082476/

Radiologist Consultation 7/20/2010

I met with the radiologist this morning for my consultation. The meeting left me feeling bummed, angry, and frustrated. I'm unable to do the 5 day targeted radiation that I hoped to receive. After chemo is complete which will be approximately 3 months from now, I will begin daily standard radiation treatment for 5 - 7 weeks. Next step for understanding my treatment plan is to meet with the oncologist on 7/29/2010 for my chemo schedule. I expect that chemo will begin either the 1st or 2nd week of August.
Warning: You may want to keep your distance from me today.

Aetna approved 7/21/2010

It is amazing what a nice, nasty letter will do. Yes, I drafted a letter and sent it to both Aetna & my HR department regarding my frustration and their incompetence. Now, I've received so many phone calls from them over the last two days it is not even funny. I even know when I receive future calls. Why do we have to go there to get action? I'm scheduled to return to work on Aug. 2nd because the maximum time allowed for a lumpectomy is 3 weeks. Here is the crazy part, I will begin chemo approximately one week later and will be out of the office again and starting the process all over.

Difficult Day 7/21/2010

Today, I'm having discomfort in my neck and chest thanks to the Port-A-Cath. As long as I'm sitting around doing nothing then I feel fine. The minute I start doing things again then I'm back down. I feel like I'm on a roller coaster ride - up and down. The thought of being stuck with this port for the next year is not sitting well with me. I'm reassured by others that it will get better. I sure hope they are all right. I'm going to have to take some drugs tonight. I've never smoked weed before but if this pain doesn't stop that might change real soon. Got you! Only kidding, I'm going to pop an Aleve. Good night!

Rough Night 7/22/2010

Last night was rough. I took 2 Aleve pills and that did nothing for my pain. The only thing I can attribute to causing the pain was my cleaning the kitchen & washing dishes. So I'm back to sitting around today which is driving me crazy. I'm so used to being active and everyone knows that I'm slightly OCD. I will must cook dinner but other than that I plan to take it easy.

~ Yes, I might be in pain but at least I'm not paralyzed. Optimism
  always ~ Leslie Michelle

Picture & details of my port 7/23/2010

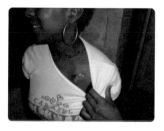

I have received many questions regarding what a Port-a-Cath is so I thought what better way to explain it than to show you a picture. I'll begin by saying that the brown, shiny spots you see on my neck and chest is actually the surgical glue that will fall off in about 3-4 weeks after surgery. The actual incision is a very small line underneath the glue. The top incision around my neck is where the catheter is inserted into my jugular vein. The catheter is connected to the port which is the "bump" or cystlike structure sticking out at the bottom incision point. The port has a septum from which drugs can be injected or blood drawn with less pain than a needle stick. The Port-a-Cath provides the benefits of preventing your veins from getting burned out as well as less discomfort. As you can see, the port is completely inserted underneath the skin with nothing protruding. Before each chemo treatment, a numbing cream is rubbed on top of the skin where the port is placed. Then a needle is stuck through the skin into the port. A saline solution is used to flush the port then treatment begins. Chemo meds are run through the port through the same needle. Nurses love this device because it eliminates the stress of trying to find a vein. Patients love the device because it is less discomfort, only one needle stick, and a lower risk of infection. I hope this demystifies the port-a-cath. If I find someone willing to video record my initial chemo treatment then I will definitely post it.

Return to church 7/25/2010
Today I returned to church and sat in my assigned seat with my crew. LOL - Yes, I'm one of those who arrive 30 minutes early so I can get the same seat up close. It was nice to see my posse again although I was afraid someone was going to hit my port with all the hugs. One of our associate ministers preached today and her sermon was titled, Stop Worrying, Start Living! Such a powerful message. I have always tried to live my life according to this principle, Live Full / Die Empty. Philippians 4:6-7 "Do not be anxious about anything, but in everything, by prayer and petition, with thanksgiving, present your requests to God. And the peace of God, which transcends all understanding, will guard your hearts and your minds in Christ Jesus."

~ Always Live Now! Enjoying all that the present moment has to offer you. Yesterday will not return and tomorrow may never arrive. ~ Leslie Michelle

Dental Appointment 7/27/2010
Today I went to my 6months checkup in preparation for chemo. I received a special prescription for toothpaste and mouth wash which is recommended for chemo patients. Apparently, the chemo meds and radiation have a tendency to dry out your mouth eliminating the much needed saliva which helps prevent cavities. By using the special toothpaste, mouth wash, & chewing gum, it will help to stimulate saliva thus providing protection for my teeth. I hate chewing gum. I've always felt that it is the nastiest invention. It is often abused by people who seem to enjoy making irritating popping noises and it is often left where others can step on it. Yuck! One of my pet peeves.

14

Confession time: I have to drive pass the only Krispy Kreme in Richmond to get to my dentist office. Yes, on my way home, I stopped and bought a dozen of glazed donuts. It has been many years since I've indulged in this pleasure. Nice!

Thursday Morning Mom 7/27/2010

I received a surprising phone call during dinner tonight. Back in May of this year, a friend nominated me for the title of Thursday Morning Mom on the national radio broadcast, Tom Joyner Morning Show. The show receives thousands of nominations & I won! Tune into the show on Thursday, July 29th to hear my spotlight. Perfect timing - I can use the money for back to school shopping for my crew It's strange being recognized and appreciated for doing what I'm supposed to do. Thank You for recognizing my efforts and being so thoughtful!

.

3 CHEMOTHERAPY

Oncologist Visit 7/29/2010

Today I had my initial oncologist consult. The doctor was hilarious and the staff great. I will have 6 doses of the chemo meds Taxotere & Carboplatin followed by Herceptin for 12 months. This is commonly referred to as TCH. I have also agreed. to be a part of a new clinical trial being sponsored by Dr. Slamon the creator of the wonder drug Herceptin. The clinical trial is known as the ALTTO Protocol. This is an international program in which I will also be given the medication referred to as Tykerb. I'm so blessed to have the best doctors on the planet. Over the next 2 weeks, I will have tons of paperwork and doctor appointments in preparation for chemo. We expect to begin the chemo meds the week of Aug. 16th. Now that I have bored you with all the medical jargon, here is the funny part of my visit. My doctor informed me that it is important to maintain a healthy sex life while on chemo. (I will not get into the graphic details of why. LOL) After I informed her that I was single and there is NO SEX going on here, my doctor gave me this goofy grin and said, "Well there is more than one way to have sex you know." Then she proceeded to give me examples. It was hilarious! As you can see none of my appointments are without entertainment. Thanks for the many cards, flowers, dinners, emails, and laughs over the last few weeks. Love You All

Appointments scheduled 7/30/2010

Back to the Oncologist today to complete a pile of consent forms. Yes, I agree to the treatment blah, blah, blah. Yes, I recognize that this medication will kill cancer cells but may also stop my heart, cause excessive tearing, dry skin, mouth sores, diarrhea, fatigue, and loss of appetite. We scheduled tons of appointments for lab work and exams which are required prior to receiving the initial chemo treatment on Aug. 19th. Chemo will occur every 3 weeks for a total of 6 treatments. The day before each treatment, I will have to repeat the full round of lab test / blood work as a precautionary step. Some of the things that will be checked is my heart and my white blood cells count.

Why is it Taboo? 8/3/2010

I have never understood why certain things are considered taboo in the African American community. We are very secretive about our health as well as our finances. This makes no sense at all. How can you help someone else if you keep your mouth closed? I'm not sure if this is specific to just my race because I've been black my whole life. But, this is something that we definitely must change. Every doctor I have encountered has been pleasantly surprised that I found the lump myself, acted so quickly, and that I have a living will as well as long-term care insurance. When I invested in these financial instruments, I did so because it was so cheap when you are young and healthy. I never imagined that I would have a need to use any of these things but it didn't make sense not to buy them at such a reasonable rate. I'm so happy that so many of you have begun to do self-exams, scheduled mammograms, and are considering a different form of exercise, belly dancing. My request: Keep up with your health and financial maintenance the same way you keep up with your car, hair, & nails. Ouch! I'm sure that will hurt some of you but medicine can be painful at times.

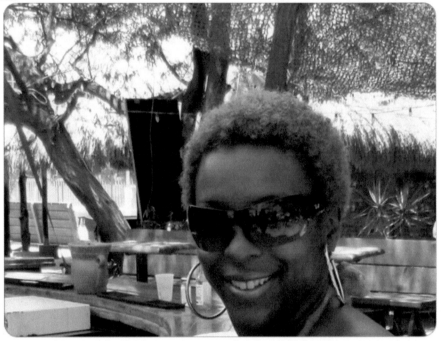

EKG 8/4/2010
Preparation begins. Today I had my baseline EKG performed. The technician took tons of pictures of my heart via Ultrasound. I will have to repeat this test approx. every 3 months to make sure that the chemo medications are not causing any damage. I was told that I have a beautiful heart - it is very photogenic. LOL. I thought the woman was crazy but she said that they are not able to capture quality pictures from many. This exam took about 30 minutes, and I was a little nervous because I was fearful that she was going to accidentally hit my port.

CT Scan 8/5/2010
Another test completed. In preparation for the CT Scan I had to refrain from eating or drinking anything after midnight last night. I had an IV with contrast (dye) run through my veins while the images were captured. That is the weirdest feeling. When the contrast begins to enter your vein, it is really cool and then followed by a hot flash. You literally feel like you have to urinate and extremely hot all over. Weird. While I was in the waiting room, another family entered and it was obvious from the scar on her chest (typical location of a port) that the wife was a cancer survivor. She sat next to me and over eagerly began to

talk about her anal cancer. WHAT? I never knew such a thing existed. So today, I'm counting my blessings - Thank God I do not have anal cancer.

Preparing for Chemo 8/8/2010

In addition to the numerous doctors' appointments, I've spent this past week preparing for Chemo. There is a lot to consider and plan for. I purchased my prescription toothpaste, medicated chewing gum & mouthwash, head scarves just to name a few. I've also been eating everything under the moon - lobster, Mexican, sushi, crab cakes, bread pudding, peach cobbler, molten lava cake and the list goes on and on. For entertainment, I've been spending time with my dear friends for dinner and enjoying jazz. I LOVE music as it is my ultimate therapy. Today's message from church was "I'm a Piece of Work - You are a Masterpiece created by God". It was an AMAZING sermon that focused on the importance of accepting all that you are and walking into your destiny. Thought for today: Just as I have been purchasing things that I need to help with my chemo journey there are also some things that I'm getting rid of. This includes not only personal belongings but people as well. Some people need you in their lives simply so that they can feel needed. Those things that do not provide me any value or are simply occupying space have been disregarded. I've become even more aware of how precious my time is and how I choose to spend it.

Surgery Bills 8/9/2010

Today I received the first two bills for my surgery. Wow! Wow! Wow! There are so many doctors and laboratories involved it is extremely difficult to keep up with it all. I'm so thankful that I have a big corporation behind me to assist in paying these medical expenses - without insurance I could not afford to be sick. With insurance, it is still a big pill to swallow. I have no clue how much each chemotreatment will cost. It looks like this may be the first time that I will be able to itemize my medical expenses on my income taxes.

Flu Shot 8/11/2010

On Monday, I took the kids to the pediatrician for a flu shot and today I received the shot as well. Typically, this is something that I would not do but under these circumstances, I felt it was wise. I'm trying to take all precautionary measures before beginning chemo.

Follow-up with Surgeon 8/13/2010

Today was my follow-up visit with my surgeon. She walked in the room eagerly telling me about a phone call that she had with a surgeon who has invented an alternative method for inserting the Port-a-Cath in your upper arm. She thanked me for providing her the information regarding this procedure and said she would let me know if I change the way she does surgeries in the future. Knowledge sharing is powerful! I have a friend, Leslie, who had a similar procedure done which prompted my research on this topic. My wounds have all healed amazingly well. She also performed an ultrasound of my breast which showed that there is no excess fluid. Everything looks good.

Lab Work 8/16/2010

Today I had all of my lab work completed for my initial chemo dose which is scheduled for this Thursday. I also spent time with a chemo nurse discussing all of the precautions that should be taken as well as warning signs. Even for someone as organized as I am, this is overwhelming. Tons of information, appointments at various locations, and medication. I have compiled a consolidated document to share with my mom. I have to make sure that there is another adult who knows what is going on and what I'm taking. The mandatory medications that I will be taking are: Taxotere, Carboplatin, Herceptin, Decadron, & Neulasta. I purchased the Walgreens prescription card in hopes that it will help cover some of the costs not picked up by my insurance. After I left the doctor, I picked up a temporary handicap decal from the DMV.

Randomized results 8/16/2010

Just received some wonderful news. When you sign up for a clinical trial, your statistics are entered into a database, and you are randomly selected for one of the arms of the trial. In the ALTTO trial that I have volunteered to participate in, there are 4 arms of study. I was selected for arm 4 which means that I get to take an additional pill known as Tykerb as well as being allowed to begin my Herceptin meds at the same time as chemo. What this means in plain English is that I get to take parallel treatments simultaneously. The tykerb is a new wonder drug that is not fully released yet. I'm so excited that I got the drugs that I wanted and also that I will be used as a vessel to further along treatment options for others who have HER2 breast cancer. God is good!

Attitude is Everything 8/17/2010

A friend sent me this poem because it reminded her of me. I hope you enjoy it as much as I did.

Attitude
There once was a woman who woke up one morning, looked in the mirror, and noticed she had only three hairs on her head.
'Well,' she said, 'I think I'll braid my hair today.'
So she did and she had a wonderful day.
The next day she woke up, looked in the mirror and saw that she had only two hairs on her head.
'H-M-M,' she said, 'I think I'll part my hair down the middle today.'
So she did and she had a grand day.
The next day she woke up, looked in the mirror and noticed that she had only one hair on her head.

'Well,' she said, 'today I'm going to wear my hair in a pony tail.'
So she did, and she had a fun, fun day.
The next day she woke up, looked in the mirror and
noticed that there wasn't a single hair on her head.
'YAY!' she exclaimed. 'I don't have to fix my hair today!'
Attitude is everything
Author unknown.

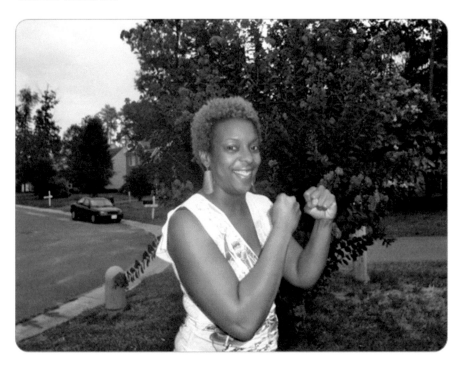

Pre-Chemo meds begin 8/18/2010

As they say in the boxing ring, Let's get ready to rumble! The day before and the day after each chemo injection, I have to take Decadron. This is a steroid that helps to prevent nausea and vomiting. Two pills at 9 am & two pills at 5 pm. During the actual chemo injections, I will be given additional medication to help prevent nausea. My Mom is arriving today and will take me to my appointments on Thursday & Friday. Hopefully, I will not have to tranquilize her. LOL

Thought: I just bought an all-natural line of makeup and now I'll go buy something cute to wear to chemo. I'm not being vain, but I do believe that you can lift your spirits by liking what you see on the outside. You must be in tune with your Mind, body, & soul. You should feel good about what you put in your body, on your body, and those that you keep around your body. It's good for the soul~ Leslie Michelle

The Big Shave 8/18/2010

I woke up this morning and decided that I would shave my hair off rather than waiting for the chemo meds to take it off. Nope - didn't discuss it with anyone because I didn't want a second opinion. Yes, I realize that I might be the 1% that doesn't lose their hair, but I choose not to be bothered with styling it during this time. I LOVE my new look.

Chemo dose#1 8/19/2010

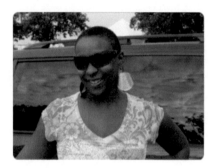

The receptionist was puzzled that I was waiting for the injection room. Guess, I did not look the part. LOL - My chemo session was from 10:00 am - 3:45 pm. I was anxious about accessing the port as I did not know what to expect. The nurse used a freezing spray to numb the area and the shot was painless. After the shot, there was a slight burning sensation that lasted for about 15 minutes. I was given 7 drugs: Tylenol, Benadryl, Aloxi, Tykerb, Herceptin, Taxotere, and carboplatin. Because I don't typically take any medication, this concoction made me extremely sleepy. I was out for about an hour during the procedure. After chemo, Mom & I went to Tripps for lunch/dinner - lobster, steak, broccoli, sweet, mashed potatoes, & water. You all know how much I love to eat so I thought I would get it all in before the nausea shows up.

White blood cells 8/20/2010

Today I returned to the doctor to receive a shot of Neulasta. It stimulates the growth of your white blood cells. This one was painful - it burned. I will have to repeat this drill every 3 weeks after each Chemo dose. I'm feeling well just extremely thirsty, so I've been trying to stay hydrated. I also have a low energy level but not too bad.

Body aches 8/21/2010

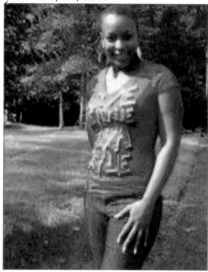

Today the sore muscles are starting to settle in, similar to the flu. Also, my bones are aching. This is caused by the injection that I had yesterday to stimulate the growth of my white blood cells.

Physically: My energy level is low.

Mentally: I could dance across the moon.

Spiritually: I feel blessed.

Soreness 8/22/2010

Last night the soreness really began to set in. The pressure of my body hurts to touch the mattress while laying down. It hurts to put a purse on my shoulder. It feels as though I have just walked away from a car accident. My mouth is constantly dry from the drugs so I'm constantly drinking water or chewing a medicated gum, biotene. My appetite remains good although I'm careful about what I'm consuming. Foods I'm trying to avoid are dairy products, spicy foods, and fried or greasy foods. I was able to attend church this morning, but the ordeal wore me out. I've been sleeping all day. I'm so thankful that I have not experienced nausea, vomiting, or stomach issues.

My throat 8/23/2010

My throat is very sore. I knew I had to avoid spicy foods, but I never considered black pepper spicy. Lord, I'm craving some Texas Pete so bad. LOL. I'm constantly freezing, and the AC makes my body ache. Guess, I'm going to have to adjust the thermostat and my sleepwear.

Cravings 8/24/2010

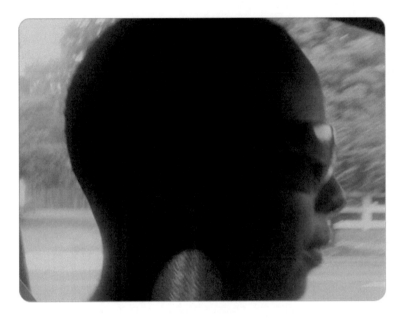

I'm having strong pregnancy-like cravings for my favorite candy, Turtles (the Original, DeMets), lobster, & Salt n Vinegar potato chips. I know these things don't go together but can't shake it. This is insane! I'm not sure that any of these foods can get down my throat but I'm going to try the candy. I learned today that I cannot have any pepper at all on my food. It causes my throat to feel as though it is closing. Very painful!

Acid Reflux 8/25/2010

Severe acid reflux today. I had to call my oncologist to find out what over-the-counter medications were safe to take. It occurs regardless of what I eat and is very painful. Praying it will not keep me up all night. Tomorrow I will be going for my next Herceptin infusion.

Herceptin treatment 8/26/2010

Today, I went to have my weekly Herceptin infusion. I was given medication for acid reflux through my port as well as a prescription drug to take daily. After treatment, I slept most of the day from the Benadryl. I've got to increase my fluid & calorie intake - I've lost 8lbs since last week.

Toenails 8/28/2010
The first visible side effect of the Herceptin showed up today. Some of my toenails are beginning to come off. The funny thing is I initially thought my polish was chipped. Guess, I will not have any need to go to my biweekly pedicures for a while. Maybe, I'll trade them in for a body massage.

Sore Head 8/30/2010
My scalp is really sore, and it is driving me crazy! Most of the folks on this medication will lose all of their hair somewhere between days 14 - 17, which is this week for me. Today, my appetite returned, and I could actually taste my food. Chemo causes your taste buds to be off - it is hit or miss depending on what you eat.

Treatment continues 9/3/2010
Yesterday, I had my 3rd Herceptin treatment. I'm beginning to feel like a pro at this. I met with both the Chemo nurse & my research nurse. The research nurse must approve my ability to continue with treatment after reading the stats on my blood work before each infusion. He documented the symptoms that I'm showing which are dark spots on my tongue and toenails which are splitting. The nurse said that he had never seen anyone with their nails split horizontally. See Mom, "I am special always" LOL

Shedding 9/7/2010
My hair has started shedding so I'm very glad that I cut most of it off. It is rather annoying to have my hair constantly on my shirt. I'm beginning to feel back to normal again, so I cooked a huge dinner for Labor Day - steaks, chicken wings, smoked sausages, jalapeno rice, broccoli & mushroom kabobs, & seafood salad. But now it is time for my next Chemo dose. I have a week full of my appointments & the kids have returned to school. The positive is that now I know what to expect when going for my chemo treatment as well as how to take care of the side effects. The negative is that I know what to expect and I'm dreading it all.

Food for Thought:1 out of 3 women has breast cancer. Most women do not discover this until it has spread throughout their body. Almost daily, I come across someone who has been impacted by this dreadful disease.

Lab Work - Chemo#2 9/8/2010
Today I'm back on steroids and completed my lab work for Chemo#2. Stats look good but starting to look slightly anemic so guess I will eat some oysters tonight! Chemo#2I'm blogging from my chemo chair. One of my besties,

Marlon took me to my Chemo#2 session today. Yes, I was a little nervous about this. For everyone who knows Marlon and how animated he is, I wasn't sure that the Cancer Center could handle it. LOL. Of course, Marlon wanted to stay with me so he could take pictures of me falling asleep with my mouth open and post the pictures online, but I reminded him that I have ammunition that he didn't want me to use against him.

~ I'm Thankful for all of my wonderful family members & friends who have selflessly offered & delivered on assisting me in many ways. Especially Mom, Shana, Hiliary, Sharon, LaMonica, Andre, Moni, Greg, Marlon, Marjorie, & Mrs. Jones for delivering cooked meals and taking time off their jobs to help with transportation to appointments. THANK YOU all. I appreciate the LOVE you have shown. ~ Leslie Michelle

First Night – Chemo#2 9/10/2010
The first Night went well. I began my chemo ritual yesterday by drinking water constantly and eating yogurt once a day. This helps flush the kidneys and keep your urinary tract healthy. I woke up several times throughout the night because my tongue and throat were throbbing. I'm trying to avoid taking any pain meds, but we will see how it goes. Because chemo compromises your immune system, I'm being extra careful by staying away from crowds, frequent use of hand sanitizers, and wearing gloves when using household cleaning products that are loaded with toxins. My son's first football game of the season is tonight. I'm trying to decide whether I should attempt to attend. Living in an air bubble is extremely difficult! Some of you have asked if I can drink alcohol while on chemo. Science or doctors do not have a definitive answer on this topic. But I chose to avoid alcohol during this time because my kidneys are already working overtime & alcohol causes dehydration which is already a symptom of the chemo medications. I will chat with you again later today after my doctor's appointment. Be Blessed!

Neulasta Shot#2 9/10/2010
Completed my Neulasta shot to stimulate my white blood cells today. This is always done the day after my chemo treatment. The first time I got this shot it burned like crazy when the medicine entered my body. However, today I had a pleasant surprise. The chemo nurse took the medication out of the fridge and allowed it to get to room temperature before I arrived as she thought it would not burn as badly. To my surprise, it did not burn at all. Small pleasures! Now I'm home recuperating. BTW - The football coach has agreed to allow me to borrow the video coverage from each game over the weekends so I can catch Triston's football season without being exposed to the high school germs. I'm excited about this!

Like Clockwork 9/11/2010

It's the 3rd night after chemo and the steroids are beginning to wear off now. This means all of the flu-like symptoms are here. Sore muscles, sore throat, & aching bones. I think I may stay home from church tomorrow. I'm trying to be careful about limiting my exposure to germs. My oldest daughter, Ashlynn, is heaven-sent. She goes out of her way to make sure that I have everything I need. She is wise beyond her years. I Thank God for this gift.

Own your health 9/12/2010

As you all know, I have to get blood work before each chemo dose. This week I made a 2nd request that the medical team check for any deficiencies I may have in any vitamin levels that could be tested. I had already begun taking Vitamin D, 2000 u per day just as a safety precaution. Well, surprise, surprise! This morning, I received an automated phone call from my local pharmacy that my prescription was ready. I was confused because I didn't recall turning in a prescription. I soon discovered that my Vitamin D level is extremely low, and my doctor called in a prescription for 50,000 u of Vitamin D to be taken once a week. Although I've been in bed all day I got up and picked up the prescription.

"Your health is your health! Don't assume that the doctors are automatically checking for anything. Ask questions & make the appropriate request. Own your health! After all, you just might save your own life". ~ Leslie Michelle

Balding 9/13/2010

Today my hair has been falling out at a rapid rate. When I noticed it, I started laughing. I think it is funny. I'll be glad when it is all gone so I don't have the constant hairballs all over my clothes and bed. It is annoying. I can't wait to see my children's reactions when they come home after school and notice the change from this morning.

In Bed 9/15/2010

I've been in bed most of the day dealing with stomach cramps & itching. I hope I'm able to shake this off before my Herceptin treatment tomorrow. Also, after this round of chemo, I'm dealing with extreme fatigue. This laying around and taking it easy is driving me crazy but I don't have the energy to do much of anything.

Treatment Day 9/16/2010

Another treatment completed! I reviewed my lab stats with the chemo nurse today. My hemoglobin count has received a slight decrease throughout the weeks. If this continues then I will need a blood transfusion. I'm not sure how I feel about this so I might ask my sisters to send me some of their blood. After treatment, I'm pretty much wiped out. I spent the remainder of the afternoon sleeping.

Why Testify? 9/17/2010

It has been almost 3 months since my diagnosis and what a journey it has been. I cannot tell you how many people I have come across who are impacted by breast cancer. The number is too numerous to count. For those of you who are still afraid to do self-exams, I would like to share some news with you. After creating this blog, 2 people have directly contacted me because they have taken my advice and discovered that they have breast cancer. In addition, my family had another scare with this disease. I urged my mother and sisters to demand a mammogram & testing for the gene known to be linked to breast cancer. Mom & Shana both had a mammogram & an MRI. Then I received a dreadful call from my sister, Shana. The test indicated that she had a cyst in one of her breasts & two cysts in the other. The doctor felt that one of the lumps was suspicious & scheduled a biopsy. We decided to not share this information with my parents or baby sister, Hiliary, until we knew for sure what we were dealing with. Shana, Chad(brother-in-law), & I were in deep prayer and complete shock over the last two weeks waiting for the exam and results. THANK GOD - the cyst was benign. People, this is real and too many are discovering this illness too late. Do not rely completely on your doctors or technology. At times the mammogram is misread or does not indicate that the disease is present. Listen to your instincts, it is given to you by God. If something doesn't seem right, look right, smell right, or if you just have an unsettling gut feeling - this is God speaking to you. Take Action!

 "Today, I'm thanking God for giving me a voice & choosing me to educate, encourage, & motivate others". ~ Leslie Michelle

A Letter From a Friend 9/17/2010

THIS IS A MUST READ!!!!!!!!! I received this email from a dear friend. I asked her if I could share it with others. I was going to condense it but do not want to remove anything important, so this is a direct quote. The only thing I will withhold is her name. (Linda is my mom)
   "Hi Linda,
   I have been putting this off now for some time, plus not having
   the energy to type this letter to you. I was devasted to initially
   learn of Leslie's Breast Cancer. I am so glad she decided to do this
   website, she may have saved my life. I had been going for my
   mammogram and several times I had to go back for diagnostics
   within six months. I question Roper St Francis Health Center
   several time and she assured me if there was anything to be
   concerned about they would have me back in their facilities in

no time. I didn't have a lump in my right breast but it was very, very firm with noticeable changes. I needed to make an appointment for my pap smear, so that's also when I requested a breast exam, this exam was the day after my birthday on the 16th of July. The physician said I should have an exam with a surgeon. They would contact me regarding the appointments. On the 5th of August, I was at the MUSC Hollings Center for a diagnostic mammogram and ultrasound, upon completion of those two exams it was determined I needed an ultra-sound guided biopsy, which can be done on the same day because they had an opening. They told me they would probably have results by Monday afternoon. However, Dr Cole called me Friday, August 6th by 5pm. and told me I had breast cancer. I know I don't have to tell you how I felt about that news. This led to several similar to Leslie, MRI< CT scan, Bone Scan, Lab work, etc. Linda, I am not going to bore you with a whole bunch of details, but I do want you to know with the MRI that led to an ultrasound and biopsy on my left breast one growth as a cyst and the other was not. The oncologist said it was a different type of cancer in each breast. The surgeon and I have already discussed that I would have to have a mastectomy on the right breast but now I think it will be both. I have already had my port placed and received my first chemo treatment which was on the 8th of September and also my Neulasta shot, the following day. I am scheduled for chemo every other week for a total of 8 injections and looking at surgery early next year. Through God all things are possible, and that he will truly bring both of us through this and well. I hope you will share this with Leslie for me. I know that she was someone the Lord placed in my life years ago, thank you for having such a lovely daughter.

I have since gotten more updates on her and her family has a history of breast cancer. Please no more secrets. Let us help each other live. She said her grandmother who raised her had breast cancer and she never knew. I have not named her but please include her in your prayers!

Side Effects 9/19/2010

I've been exhausted over the last week and I'm not doing anything except lying in bed. I developed a UTI exactly 8 days after chemo#1 & #2. Both times I was placed on an antibiotic to clear up the infection. I've also been having a difficult time trying to force myself to eat. I have not had much of an appetite over the last few days. I'm lucky if I can get one meal down so I've been living off of Ensure and fruit smoothies. At times my thoughts are not clear, and I am forgetful, this is often referred to as chemo brain. Today, I find myself

wondering, is it worth it to go through this treatment. I know the answer is yes, but I completely understand why so many others opt not to endure
this plan. This too shall pass. I'm looking forward to the day that this will be behind me, and I will be having the chemo-is-over party.

Morning Joy 9/20/2010
After going to bed at 6 pm last night and not waking until 6:30 am this morning, I'm feeling much better. I didn't even know I could sleep that long. Today is the first day in about a week that I have not awakened to stomach cramps, and I was able to eat breakfast. Today is a good day.

Funny start today 9/21/2010
I woke up this morning and jumped out of bed. I heard a ding sound as if something hit the hardwood floor. I immediately knew what it was without even looking. But I looked anyway. Yes, one of my toenails had fallen off. Another side effect of my chemo drugs. Hilarious

Cocktail party 9/23/2010
Getting ready for my weekly Herceptin cocktail party. Me with my 9 toenails, black spotted tongue, bald head, and crazy sense of humor. LOL - Got to find joy in everything because God is good! I'm enjoying a little Will Downing this morning. His new CD is amazing. I thought I would share one of the songs, "Consensual" https://www.youtube.com/watch?v=FadBXl6Uics. Hope you enjoy it. Have a Blessed Day!

The Weekend is Here 9/24/2010
The treatment went well yesterday. I slept most of the day after returning home. Today, I'm still tired. I will get some rest this weekend as I prepare for next week which will be the halfway point. Priceless: Andre, my neighbor, took me to treatment yesterday. When I told the chemo nurse that a toenail fell off, you should have seen the look of shock/disbelief on his face. It was priceless!
I wish I had caught it on camera.

Living in the present 9/28/2010

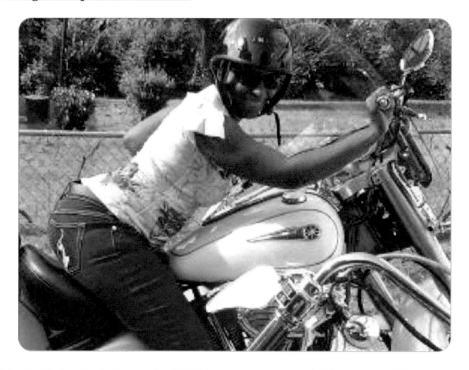

No, I didn't take it for a spin BUT I sure was tempted. This cancer thing is forcing me to be cautious and limiting my ability to be spontaneous. So, I opted to take a Biker Chick photo and leave it at that. This week will be my halfway point for my chemo treatment - that's right Chemo#3. I have a week full of appointments beginning Wednesday & I'm praying that all of my stats are looking good so nothing is delayed.

"Enjoy the present. Don't gamble on waiting for the kids to be grown, or that special birthday, or monumental anniversary. Those things are special too but live a little now. I sure do." ~ Leslie Michelle

Prep for Chemo#3 9/29/2010
All of the fun for round#3 begins today. Back on the steroids & to the doctor for lab work. Praying that all of my numbers are right so I can continue with my treatment course. I received a call yesterday from my research nurse and she indicated that they may have to reduce the levels of my meds since I lost a toenail. I told her that I'm good, it allows me to save money at the spa on my pedicures. LOL

Approved for Chemo#3 9/29/2010

I got my approval to receive Chemo#3 tomorrow. My stats indicate that I'm now anemic so that explains the lingering fatigue and long naps I'm taking daily. I picked up a multi-vitamin and will have to eat some beef which I have been avoiding since treatment began. Prayerfully, I will enjoy the taste. The doctor has recommended that I return to work on Jan. 2nd. Hopefully, the insurance company will not give me any drama because I don't have the energy to fight these days. Wow - I can't believe that I said that I don't have the energy to fight. I should have kept that to myself because I don't want anyone to take advantage of me. LOL

Headed to Chemo#3 - 9/30/2010
I'm headed to Chemo#3 - Wow, this is the halfway point for the Big Bad Drugs. I'm so excited. I bought some cute breast cancer cupcakes for the chemo nurses. I want them to know that they are appreciated. I've been told that I look good, and it is hard to believe that I'm going through this journey. Here is my secret: Well, I don't think I should let cancer steal my spirit. It already has my freedom, my time, my health, my hair, my energy, my nails, my Cîroc, & my Grey Goose. So, I refuse to let anything, or anyone steal my spirit, EXCEPT God. Talk to you soon.

Chemo#3 complete! - 9/30/2010
Chemo#3 COMPLETE. The chemo nurses enjoyed the cupcakes. They work super hard to make sure that we are all very comfortable, often foregoing lunch. What a wonderful crew! I returned home around 12:30 and went straight to bed. I was able to enjoy a wonderful dinner & now back to bed. I'm still doped up on all the meds & tomorrow will return for my injection to control my white blood cells. I'm very proud of my neighbor, LaMonica. She mastered multi-tasking today by taking me to treatment & having her very 1st mammogram in the same building. For those who have never had a mammogram, don't believe the crazy emails aimed to scare you. It really is not painful at all. Goodnight

Neulasta#3 complete! - 10/1/2010
I began my day by having my Neulasta injection. It burned like crazy as the meds entered my body. Fortunately, it doesn't last long. I just sit there and grit my teeth while holding my breath. I've been tired today and dealing with nausea so have been in bed all afternoon. Mentally, I feel wonderful. Just waiting for my body to catch up with my mind.

Knocked out! - 10/2/2010

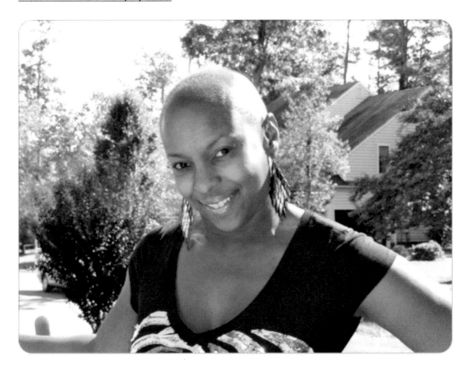

My day started pretty well with the standard side effects that I've become accustomed to - fatigue, stomach aches, and night sweats. Because it was such a beautiful day, and I felt guilty about not being able to do much with the kids I got a little adventurous. I got one of my girlfriends to accompany us to the State Fair. BIG MISTAKE! After about 1hour, I began to feel weak and told my crew that I needed to sit down. I made it to the table but not the chair before blacking out. When I woke up, I was laid out on top of the table with the EMT staff surrounding me. Lesson Learned!!! No more adventure until I'm done with this chemo. Thank God, I had an adult with me and was not driving. I'm well and back in bed. I will be calling my doctor on Monday to let her know about this event. Goodnight

Recuperating -10/3/2010

Chemo#3 has been no joke. I've been in bed ALL day. I'm still dealing with body aches and fatigue as well as pains from the fall when I passed out yesterday. I spoke to my chemo nurse today and will have to go into the office tomorrow just to make sure that my stats are okay. Staying in this house & in my bed is driving me CRAZY. And now, Vick is injured, and the Eagles are not looking so good today. Tomorrow will be better. After all, I went through to get to the state fair and guess what? The elephant ear vendors were out of

Bavarian cream. I swear it must be a conspiracy against me right now. LOL

All is well - 10/4/2010

I just returned from the doctor. The fainting spell was from dehydration and over-exertion. My platelets and red blood cells are low, but everything is okay. My red blood count is actually higher than it was after Chemo#2 which is great. My blood pressure and kidney function are normal. I was instructed to take it easy drink lots of fluids, and eat soups, potatoes, and bananas.

Another one bites the dust - 10/6/2010

Hello, I've been taking it easy. Nothing but sleeping, eating, and taking medication. Today another toenail fell off. That's right Another one bites the dust! Do you remember that song from the 80s? LOL This time I had on a pair of socks and found it floating in the bottom. Oh well, good thing it is fall and I can live in my boots for the next few months.

Treatment Thursday - 10/7/2010

It's Treatment Thursday which means infusion, lunch, & sleep. My hemoglobin is low and my magnesium level. I was instructed to eat a couple of chocolate bars, rest, and drink lots of fluids. I don't think the nurse knew who she was talking to. That sounds like music to my ears. Yesterday was a rough, rough day dealing with diarrhea. Yuck! I think it was a combination of the Starbucks and medication. I will not repeat that mistake. Back to my decaf herbal tea only.

Stomach cramps - 10/8/2010

My severe stomach cramps have continued. If this symptom doesn't improve today then I will have to stop taking the clinical trial medication, Tykerb. Some of you have tried to reach me by phone. Sorry, my energy level has been low, and I have not felt like talking. I will get caught up on the phone calls soon. What a week I have experienced!

What a week! - 10/9/2010

This has been a rough week, but I believe my stomach is beginning to settle. I have not been able to eat or drink much the last couple of days. Just my luck - I've been instructed to eat chocolate candy bars and I have not been well enough to do it. That is just plain evil! I have a Milk Chocolate Hershey's with Almonds sitting on my nightstand waiting for me to attack it. (Thanks - LaMonica!) You know it's bad when even McDonalds' Iced Tea is not appealing. I know that there are better days ahead & I look forward to them.

Things you should NEVER say - 10/10/2010

Okay, I thought I would start a list of the things you should NEVER say to a breast cancer patient. I'm dealing with hunger, fatigue, pain, etc. so some comments right now are not settling well with me. I've been VERY irritable this week and trying to save everyone from my wrath. Trust me, I understand that everyone means well but girlfriend is running out of patience these days. (I didn't have much to start with).

So here is my list:

1. You should make yourself eat/drink something "No, shit! Tell me something I don't already know!"

2. I remember when I found a lump, bump, scrape, etc. on my breast but it was nothing. "And how does this help me?"

3. Your hair will grow back, and it will be so pretty - "Who cares! And I may not want it to grow back.

Being bald is carefree and I'm enjoying it". Thanks for allowing me to release today. Can you imagine the shock I would receive if I responded to folks in the way outlined above. I think it would make a great episode of Curb Your Enthusiasm. (Expressing the thoughts that go through your head, but you just don't say them). It might be just the humor I need to get me through the day.

Today, I'm THANKFUL that I was able to eat a meal and keep it down for the first time in several days. And I'm thankful that I'm patient enough not to respond to folks with some of the thoughts that are going through my head today. LOL

Feeling better today - 10/11/2010

Thank God I've come out of my episode that started last Wednesday. I was able to eat breakfast & dinner yesterday. It felt so good to finally get some food in my system. While dealing with severe cramps, the BRAT diet seems to work best. B Bananas, R-Rice, A-applesauce, & T-toast. It is also strange that I have to pretty much avoid all of the healthy stuff that I'm accustomed to eating like whole grains, salads, fresh fruit & veggies. Right now, meat & potatoes along with multivitamins work best. I talk often to other survivors on the HER2 support forum. This site is great for sharing lessons learned on how to deal with the symptoms and researching treatment options. Knowledge is key! As common as the cold - 10/12/2010 Robin Roberts, Hoda Kotb, & Rene Syler. Do you know what these ladies have in common? Yes, they are all well-known TV anchors from each of the major networks and all are breast cancer survivors. Hoda Kotb: co-host of the Today Show Rene Syler: co-host of The Early Show from 2002 - 2007 Robin Roberts: tv anchor for the Good Morning America show This disease is no longer for older women entering menopause and coping with hormonal changes. I pray that we can figure out what is causing this rather than simply controlling it with drugs.

Treatment Thursday - 10/14/2010

I just returned from my weekly Herceptin treatment. My hemoglobin numbers continue to decrease and are dangerously low. The chemo nurse talked to me today about having a blood transfusion. They will continue to monitor me over the next week or two and make a determination. Also, I was told to stop taking my clinical trial drug, Tykerb, for 1 week to give my body a break from the harsh side effects. (Severe stomach aches / diarrhea).

Peace Be Still - 10/18/2010

I've been home taking it easy. The side effects of having a low hemoglobin count are extreme fatigue and being cold. I purchased a couple of hats to keep some of my body heat in because my head is COLD. Guess, I may have to break down and buy me a Beyonce wig - LOL. Also, I'm easily exhausted from simple things and have not been able to do any housework or cooking. Looking forward to Thursday when I will learn if I will be able to continue with my chemo treatment or not. Right now, I'm preparing for the unknown: Chemo, blood infusion, continuing with Tykerb, or medication to stimulate red blood cells. These are all of the things that are on the table right now, I'll have to wait until Thursday's blood work and consultation with my medical team to learn what course of action is next. This may sound crazy to some of you but despite all of this, I feel wonderfully at peace. Despite the distraction of breast cancer, I remain faithful to God. I think God's trying to tell me something so I'm waiting to hear his word. Matthew 8:23-27

Treatment Thursday - 10/21/2010

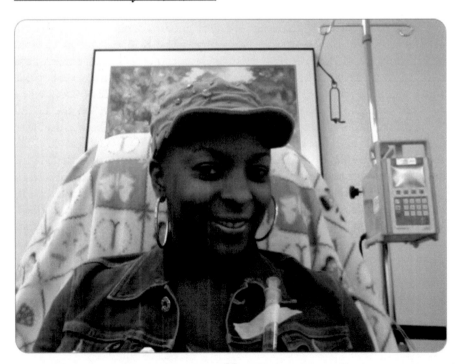

Today, I'm writing from the chemo chair. My hemoglobin only dropped from 8.7 to 8.6 which means I will be allowed to receive my 4th chemo treatment today. The overall stats look good, and my organ functions are great. God is Good! I'm also scheduled for a blood transfusion next week to get my count back into the normal range which is 12 - 15. My chauffeur today is one of my besties, Marlon, so I'm sure to be entertained. LOL Thanks for all of your encouraging words & prayers, Love You All.

Recovering from Chemo#4 - 10/22/2010

Breakfast this morning tasted like cardboard. Guess I should be used to this cycle by now but I'm not. I will be going to the doctor this afternoon to get my injection to stimulate my white blood cells. This usually kicks off the bone aches/muscle pains. What's coming up next week? On Monday afternoon, I will be going to Regional Memorial Hospital for blood typing & then on Tuesday morning, I will report to Outpatient for a blood transfusion.

Insomnia - 10/23/2010

These steroids have made me so wired that I cannot sleep. I'm sure I will crash & burn tomorrow when I'm off the pills. Thank God I only take the steroids the day before, the day of, & the day after chemo. Otherwise, I would not be a happy camper.

Muscle Aches - 10/24/2010

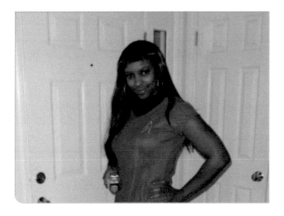

Last night my bestie, Marlon, took me to a Halloween costume party. I went as Lieutenant Uhura from Star Trek & he went as Madea. It was hilarious! It was nice to get out of the house, but I couldn't do anything but sit in a chair. There were tons of delicious food, but I was not able to eat :(The muscle aches have begun to set in & I'm exhausted! I must figure out what's for dinner today - getting tired of pizza, Chinese, & subs.

Blood Typing - 10/25/2010

Dealing with exhaustion and shortness of breath. I've spent most of the day in bed with the exception of going to get my blood typing done. I have a slight fever that we have to watch and make sure that I'm not coming down with an infection. Today, little things wipe me out like eating or trying to cook. I've been told that I will feel like a new person after the transfusion tomorrow. I can't wait for the burst of energy. I sure do need it.

Blood Transfusion - 10/26/2010

I picked up some snacks/lunch from the grocery store since I will be spending the day at the hospital. I must have looked pretty bad because the senior citizen chased me down, took my bags to the car, and shut my car door for me. I've just taken Tylenol & Benadryl, which helps control any allergic reactions that might occur. Now, I'm waiting for the blood to be sent up so that the fun can begin.

Enough! - 10/27/2010

For the last 24 hours, I've been dealing with severe stomach cramps/bloating. I will not be taking any more of the drug, Tykerb, which causes this symptom. I'm not one to complain but this is unbearable. I will consult with my medical staff tomorrow.

Treatment Thursday- 10/28/2010

What a BEAUTIFUL day! The sun is shining, and the leaves are changing. No, I'm not feeling great but I'm alive & God exists. Ready to kick this Cancer back to HELL because I have so much to do! "To my REAL friends, I'm so THANKFUL for all of your support. I will never forget your kindness and selfless acts. To my FAKE friends, I'm so THANKFUL that you have been revealed. You may exit, stage left. God Bless you all!" ~Leslie Michelle

Improving - 10/29/2010

My hemoglobin number is back up to 10.3 thanks to the transfusion. And the stomach cramps have eased up tremendously since I have come off of the Tykerb. The doctors will restart me on the Tykerb at the end of December or early January when the harsh chemo drugs have ended. I'm beginning to get a little pep in my step. Maybe, I will be up to wig shopping this weekend. I must prepare for the winter that is lurking around the corner. Ummmm what color will I be?

I'm back! - 10/31/2010

Yes! I'm able to eat again. The monster in my gut has finally quieted and the pain has stopped at last. This was a rough, rough week. Actually, the worst so far. I'm talking about constant pain that wakes you up from a sound sleep because of moaning from discomfort. I'm so glad that this episode is behind me. Racing ahead towards the chemo finish line. Two more to go!

Treatment Thursday - 11/4/2010
I don't want to go! I don't feel like going. I'm not going. - Just Kidding. LOL. Ok, my meltdown is over - I'm grabbing some breakfast and off to treatment I go. Reminder: Have your initial baseline mammogram at age 35. If there are no abnormalities and you are not deemed high risk, you will continue with annual mammograms starting at age 40.

Echo#2 - 11/8/2010
Hectic week ahead of me as I prepare for Chemo#5. I have a doctor's appointment every day this week. These copays are definitely adding up at $40 a pop. Today, I had my second Echo done. My oncologist checks on my heart every 3 months to make sure the Herceptin is not causing any damage. I'm getting excited about nearing the end of part 1, chemo. Still a long road ahead but ready for this part to be over!

Surgeon Follow-up - 11/9/2010
Today, I had my 3-month follow-up visit with my surgeon. She took an ultrasound to make sure that everything healed properly. Now, I'm at home dealing with a maintenance crew installing my new HVAC system. While performing the installation they accidentally cut my waterline - oh boy, what a day!

Chemo#5 - 11/11/2010

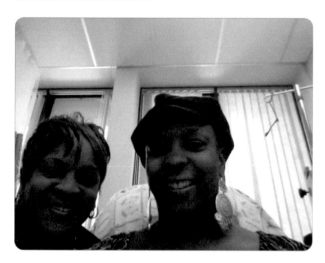

Today is Chemo#5 & my Mom came to join me for the week. I just completed my lab work and now we are waiting for the fun to begin.

Resting - 11/15/2010

I've been taking it easy as I recuperate from Chemo#5. Happy to have my mom here to assist with the little things like housework and dinner. She has been amazing as usual. My symptoms this time have been the same extreme fatigue, body aches, and sore muscles. I'm also dealing with sporadic hot flashes. I hope that the flashes disappear before I return to work, or I may be arrested for indecent exposure. LOL

Flashing - 11/16/2010

The chemo has my hormones going crazy! I've been dealing with hot flashes that send me outside in the cold with very little on to get relief. Guess it is a good thing that there is nothing behind my house except trees.

Treatment Thursday - 11/18/2010

You know it's sad when the receptionist at the doctor's office accountable for taking your money recognizes that you have a new debit card. LOL. I'm pretty exhausted today. More tired than usual. My Vitamin D level is still severely low so I'm back on 50,000 units a week.

Teeth - 11/20/2010

A new symptom has developed - my teeth are SUPER sensitive to anything remotely cold. This is making it difficult for me to get my required fluids. I keep telling myself ALMOST over - one more chemo & hopefully my body will begin to return to normal. I also have tingling or numbness in my fingers which is beginning to affect my ability to perform simple tasks like buttoning a shirt or opening items.

Numb fingers - 11/23/2010

It is becoming increasingly difficult to perform simple tasks because my fingertips are numb. I will be discussing this symptom with my medical team again tomorrow - it has to be monitored closely to avoid permanent damage. Special Thanks to my mom for coming last week and doing all the prep work to make my Thanksgiving cooking possible. It may take me longer than usual with the numb fingers and my required naps, but I will get it done.

Thankful - 11/25/2010

As usual, I slept most of the day after completing treatment yesterday. Thanksgiving is my absolute favorite holiday, and I have so much to be Thankful for - my family, friends, job, medical insurance, early diagnosis, & my testimony. I pray that I'm able to finish cooking this morning and enjoy the taste of the food today. I'm a little concerned about the numbness in my fingers because I have one more chemo next week. The doctor will determine if we need to decrease the dosage amount of the drug Taxotere because this could cause permanent damage. God is in charge - I'm not going to stress over it.

Have a Happy Thanksgiving ~Enjoy your loved ones & help someone less fortunate.

Hair - 11/28/2010

What in the world is going on? My hair is starting to grow - got a little peach fuzz appearing on my head. Not sure why this is occurring before the end of chemo. Most people don't have hair growth until 3 months after treatment. Most of the time I'm wearing a hat or wig because of the cold weather. The countdown is on to the last chemo on Thursday!

Insomnia - 11/30/2010

Insomnia has returned. I'm up most of the night & exhausted during the day. Not sure if the meds are causing this or if I'm just anxious/excited about completing the last Chemo this week. Amazingly, so many of us walk around completely unaware of some things that are going on in the world because they do not apply to our personal lives. I receive emails or phone calls at least once a week from someone who is going through treatment or just completed treatment. Before being bit by this bug, I had no clue how large this community is. Now, I find myself wondering how many of my friends/family members have this disease and are completely unaware of it. Reminder: Self-check saves lives! Feel your boobies today.

Steroids - 12/1/2010

Started my steroids this morning for Chemo#6. I'm feeling well just ready to get through tomorrow. I didn't think I would ever say this, but I can't wait to start working out again. Looking forward to the feeling returning to my fingers and toes, my energy level increasing, my toenails re-growing, and hot flashes disappearing. I've gotten a little spoiled by not having to style my hair so I'm not overly concerned about my hair growth.

The Big Day - Chemo#6 - 12/2/2010

The big day has just arrived. I haven't gone to bed yet because I'm so EXCITED. Praying that my lab work is great and that chemo#6, the Final, goes smoothly. Chemo Completed - 12/2/2010

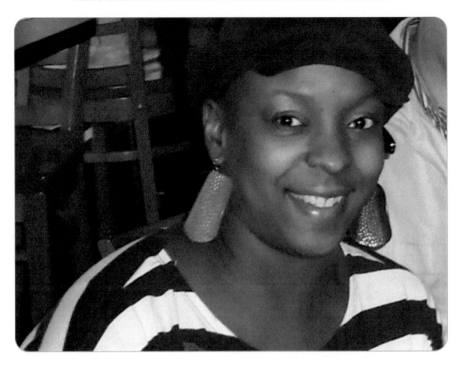

Chemo is completed! As usual, I ate lunch and then slept the rest of the day. My lab work looks pretty good although my hemoglobin number has fallen to 9.1 which means I may feel fatigued again - this should begin to recover although it will take a couple of months to restore to normal numbers. I will continue with weekly Herceptin infusions on Dec. 9th & Dec. 16th & then convert to every 3 weeks beginning January. The side effects of this drug are a cakewalk compared to chemo. Having chemotherapy behind me & being cancer-free is the best Christmas present ever!

Final Neulasta - done! - 12/3/2010
I just returned from getting my final Neulasta injection for stimulating the growth of my white blood cells. The symptoms that have begun so far from the chemo is severe hot flashes. I'm still on steroids today so I'm still medicated - the real pain begins tomorrow. "How has this experience changed me so far? I've always recognized that life is short, and you should truly enjoy each day, but I've become even more committed to this. So, watch out now! I'm going to be more spontaneous than before, I will continue my spiritual growth without failing into the traps of being religious that I have seen so many others fall cripple to, I will continue to make sure that all of my friends and family know how dear they are to me, and I will do whatever I want, whenever I want remembering to always help others when I can & take time to enjoy the present. "~ Leslie Michelle

Steroids done! - 12/4/2010

Woo Hoo - the excitement is in the air. I took my last steroids tonight. Moving forward towards the finish line. Yes, I'm dealing with fatigue, but nothing can contain my joy. "I'm feeling incredibly optimistic, vibrant, determined, encouraged, and just amazingly blessed. Thank You, God for your continuous grace and favor over my life. My strength comes from thee". ~ Leslie Michelle

Muscle Aches - 12/5/2010

What a beautiful morning! We have the first dusting of winter snow, and the sun is shining. The sore muscles and body aches began last night and are still present this morning. My fingertips are hurting & sore as well. My taste buds are distorted, and some foods are good and others I cannot taste. "Despite the pains, I'm basking in the love of my God, family & friends. I'm filled with joy. I'm truly blessed! Have a wonderful day". ~ Leslie Michelle

Healing - 12/6/2010

I spent most of yesterday in bed dealing with extreme fatigue. The side effects that I'm dealing with are itchy skin, joint pain, numb fingers, and an uncontrollable appetite. I'm starving like I'm 8 months pregnant or something. I'll be glad when the medications are out of my system so this can be under control. Also, my head is really sore again so I guess I will be losing the few follicles that have begun to grow already. LOL

Herceptin day - 12/9/2010

Good morning, friends, I'm doing well & feeling fabulous. In my mind, I could run a marathon but, in my body, I know I better wait a little while. LOL, I'm still dealing with incredible hunger. Not sure what is causing this, but I hope it corrects itself soon or I will need a new wardrobe. I'm off to my Herceptin treatment this morning & then to consult with my radiologist to sign consent forms. "Live a little today. I plan to." ~Leslie Michelle

Feeling Courageous - 12/9/2010

I was feeling a little bold today & allowed my nurse to access my port without using the freeze spray. It wasn't bad at all. After leaving my Herceptin treatment, I headed to the radiologist's office. We reviewed the treatment dos and dont's and signed the consent forms to begin treatment. Next week, I will have what is called a planning session & the daily radiation treatments will begin in January. My light is shining - 12/10/2010 Good Morning, I have this brilliant sun shining on the inside and I just can't contain it but would love to share it. So, if you see me smiling or laughing and you start to wonder if I have "completely" lost my mind the answer is not yet. "Thank You God for the incredible joy you continue to provide in my life. There is nothing like it because it is not of this world. It is not conditional. It cannot be taken away by anyone". ~Leslie Michelle

Alabaster Box - 12/11/2010

I'm a little down today because I cannot attend my son's State Championship game for high school football. My white blood cells were low, and my nurse thought it would not be a good idea. I'm trying to come down with a sinus infection, so I have taken some meds & drinking herbal tea with honey. I was listening to one of my favorite songs this morning, Alabaster Box by CeCe Winans. Wow - this song has even more meaning to me now. I LOVE this song, especially this part which had to have been written just for me: You weren't there the night He found me You did not feel what I felt When he wrapped his love all around me and You don't know the cost of the oil in my alabaster box

Gratitude - 12/12/2010

True friends who give unselfishly and expect nothing in return are RARE. There have been many who have assisted me during the last few months but few who I must mention by name. Darlene, LaMonica, Marlon, Greg, & Andre THANK YOU for grocery shopping, preparing meals, picking up medication, and transporting me and my kids wherever we needed to go. I will never forget your kindness. To show my gratitude I wanted to do something special for such a wonderful crew. Tonight, I took them to one of my favorite restaurants, Copper Grill. What a treat!

4 RADIATION

Preparing for simulation - 12/13/2010

In the morning, I will go to my simulation appointment at the Massey Cancer Center. This is the planning session to prepare for radiation treatment. During the simulation process, small tattoos that look like a freckle are placed on the breast to mark the treatment field. I've been told that it feels like an insect bite. X-rays and computer readings are reviewed to make sure that the tattoos are in the right place. Simulation is important because it helps ensure accurate positioning for the actual radiation treatment.

Simulation complete - 12/14/2010

My simulation appointment was this morning. They had me twist my body like I was a pretzel to get computer images & then hold the pose for about 5 minutes. After the initial images were taken, two small tattoos were placed on my breast. It felt like a bee sting. My sister, Shana asked me to take a picture and send it to her via text message. Of course, that would never happen for two reasons 1) I would never allow anyone to do a Brett Favre on me 2) The tattoos are unnoticeable; I can't find them. LOL

Herceptin treatment - 12/15/2010

Woo Hoo! Today is my last doctor's appointment in 2010. I moved my Herceptin appointment up a day to avoid the potential bad weather that is headed our way tomorrow. I will receive a larger dose of Herceptin because we are converting to a treatment schedule that will be once every 3 weeks.

Relaxation - 12/23/2010

Nice to have a few days without having a doctor's appointment. Even better not having to pay the copays. I'm visiting family & friends and enjoying the holiday season. My health is well but still suffering from nerve damage in my hands & feet - numbness & tingling. I'm prayerful that this is not permanent because it is driving me crazy. I'm going to take the next week off from blogging but it will start again in the new year. My daily radiation treatment begins on Jan 3rd. and runs for 7 weeks. Have a Wonderful Holiday.

Nerve damage - 12/28/2010

I've been enjoying the holidays with my family but also dealing with nerve damage in my fingers & toes. One fingernail is now separating from the nail bed. The doctor has me on medication 3 times a day which causes me to be drowsy. Also, antibiotics to prevent infection. Hope this will get better soon.

Neuropathy - 12/29/2010

I'm dealing with severe neuropathy. One of my fingernails began separating from the nail bed this week with pus oozing out & a disgusting odor. My oncologist has put me on an antibiotic & another med to assist with the nerve damage. I need help with many tasks like buttons, opening cans, & difficulty holding a pen. Now, even typing is a challenge. This will prevent me from returning to work on Monday, which is a bummer because my short-term disability ended on 12/26 & it could take up to 45 days for me to find out whether they will approve me for long-term disability. Hope this condition is temporary & that the meds will help to repair some of the damage caused by the chemo drugs.

Part II of the journey - 1/3/2011
Part II of this journey begins tomorrow, with daily radiation treatments for 7 weeks. I feel like I should have a frequent flyer card with the hospital. The neuropathy continues. What does it feel like? My fingertips are numb and extremely sensitive. Not typing much these days, having difficulty getting dressed, cleaning, & cooking. You never realize how much you use your fingertips until you try not to use them. The numb feeling in my feet is as though I've been sitting out in the cold too long or they have fallen asleep. I'm reluctantly taking the drugs that were prescribed to assist with this and hope that it will improve very soon.

First day of radiation - 1/4/2011
My first radiation appointment took about 30 minutes. It was rather uneventful just like taking an x-ray. The most difficult part of the appointment was trying to put the gown on & then trying to open the locker to get my clothes. My numb fingers made both tasks extremely difficult. 32 more treatments to go!

Hectic day - 1/5/2011
Today was hectic and tomorrow will not be much better. I met with my oncologist for a checkup & lab work. I will restart the Tykerb pills tomorrow at a higher dosage than before. This is the medication that causes severe stomach cramps & diarrhea. I will begin with the restricted BRAT diet - bananas, rice, apple sauce, & toast. I will gradually try to introduce other foods into my diet. My oncologist also increased the dosage of my medication for neuropathy. It will take a few months for this to improve. After leaving the oncologist, I went to the hospital for my second dose of radiation. I'm glad I had a break over the Christmas holiday because my schedule has returned to an insane pace.

Dear Friend - 1/5/2011
Today, I discovered that a friend was diagnosed yesterday with breast cancer. She went in for a routine annual checkup and at the end of her visit reminded the doctor that she was supposed to examine a swollen area under her arm that they were watching. The doctor decided to have a mammogram ordered and to her astonishment cancer was discovered. This young lady just like me is under 40 years of age, too young for the annual mammogram. "Dear Friend, know that I am here for you. We will get through this. I will hold your hand, attend doctor appointments, share my experiences, or just be an ear. I'm so glad that

I have documented my journey and pray that it will help you understand the road ahead of you." ~Leslie Michelle

Herceptin infusion - 1/6/2011

I'm writing from the cancer treatment center where I'm receiving my Herceptin infusion. Today, we begin a larger dosage because the new schedule will be once every 3 weeks through July. They just gave me Tylenol & the Benadryl is flowing through my veins so I'm starting to feel high. Call for self-maintenance: Don't forget to look at & feel your boobies or have someone else feel them for you. If there is a new shape, itching, lump, or color then schedule an exam right away.

First-week radiation - 1/8/2011

The first week of radiation is behind me. 6 more weeks to go! No major complications from the procedure, which is great. Still dealing with problems with my fingers and feet. Trying to take it easy and not make it worse but it is so hard. Everything requires you to use your fingers. And I am still waiting to see if Aetna will approve my LTD. I received a message this morning from another friend who has just gotten word that her mammogram is suspicious. She will have to undergo further testing to determine if it is cancer. This is crazy! Too many young folks are suffering. What is going on?

Neuropathy continues - 1/11/2011

I'm still learning to deal with this neuropathy. Earlier this week, I tried to wear a pair of my grown & sexy boots - wow, that was a mistake. I think I'm going to have to buy a pair of those ugly Naturalizer clogs or something equally disgusting. You all know how I am about my boots, so this is truly killing me. First, you take away my vodka martinis, Second, you force me to limit my chocolate intake, & now, you prevent me from wearing my boots. Damn you to hell cancer - go away from us all & never come back!

Forgive me - 1/13/2011

"Lord, forgive me for I have sinned. I bought a pair of Easy Spirit antigravity shoes". LOL - I surrender to the power of neuropathy. I cannot wear my normal shoes because my feet are extremely uncomfortable. I thought I would miraculously bounce back right after finishing the chemo drugs but that is not the case. Oh well, I will have to take baby steps instead of running. "I can see the sun peaking from behind the mountain. Better days are near". ~ Leslie Michelle

Exhaustion - 1/15/2011

Yesterday, I reached a whole new level of exhaustion. After my radiation treatment, I was pretty much sleepwalking. I left the treatment room, passed the dressing room, entered the lobby, and got to the exit door before realizing that I failed to put my clothes on. LOL - That's right, I was still in my hospital gown. Thank God, I only get undressed from the waist up and that it is winter. The cold air woke me up. The technician was concerned about me driving home but I called my sister who stayed on the phone with me during my drive. Hope I will be able to get some much needed rest this weekend.

Out of commission - 1/18/2011

I wanted a home cook meal tonight but that was a mistake. My fingers didn't like the work and started bleeding. Looks like I will have to refrain from cooking until my fingers heal. Bummed! Good thing I don't have any hair right now because I wouldn't be able to fix it.

Neuropathy continues - 1/23/2011

My fingers are killing me, so I have not been blogging as often. I was up all night with throbbing pains in my finger. Tylenol PM has given me some relief. Hopefully, this will heal pretty soon.

Busy Day! - 1/25/2011

It has been a hectic day with multiple doctor appointments. There is nothing more the doctors can do about the nerve damage, so they gave me some legalized cocaine, in other words hydrocodone to help with the pain. So I guess, the answer is keep me doped up & in bed until my fingers begin to heal. Off to La-La land I go!

Throbbing - 1/29/2011

The throbbing pain in my finger is finally easing up. Not sure if it is getting better or the meds are just keeping me high. Either way I'm happy for the relief. Advice: For those coming though chemo with the drug, Taxotere keep your nails cut as short as possible throughout treatment. The nails tend to separate from the nail bed and become very sensitive after treatment is over. No one told me this, so I wasn't prepared.

What is radiation like? - 2/7/2011

I have not been blogging as often these days because my fingers have been bleeding. Radiation is going well & I can see the finish line - 25 out of 33 completed. 8 more treatments to go! I'm often asked "What is radiation like?" It is completely painless - a laser shines down on you just like taking a picture. What are the side effects? Fatigue, darkening of the skin, & itching.

5 Boosters left - 2/11/2011

Today I completed my 28 days of general radiation to the entire breast. I have 5 more days left of what is called a booster dose which is to a small, targeted area only. I'm so excited!!!!

Insurance - 2/16/2011

Surprise, surprise. After several calls to Aetna & Capital One over the last two months and speaking to numerous reps to ensure that my medical coverage remains intact, it is screwed up. Wish I could say that I'm surprised but I'm not. I received a COBRA insurance bill today for $1500 (single coverage) and they dropped my kids off my insurance. So now I have the pleasure of trying to speak with someone knowledgeable enough to get all of this mess corrected.

Yesterday - 2/18/2011

Yesterday I had my Herceptin treatment and took a girlfriend with me. I wanted her to see what the infusion center experience was like as she will begin chemo on March 24th for breast cancer. I also went to a dermatologist to see what could be done about my fingers. That was a complete waste of my $40 and time. The doctor advised me to cut my nails short, keep them clean, and just let them grow out. Dah! Tell me something I don't already know. Oh well, I did what my oncologist suggested.

Radiation complete! - 2/18/11

Radiation treatment: 7 weeks (33 rounds) Monday - Friday is officially DONE. I'm so glad to have this chapter behind me. I will continue with the Tykerb pills daily & Herceptin every 3 weeks until the end of July. Thank You for all of your prayers & support.

Frustrated w/ fingers - 2/19/11

Yucky finger trauma lingers on. The dermatologist said it could take 4 - 6 months before it improves. This is extremely frustrating, every little thing I attempt to do starts the fingers to bleed. I was given a steroid & antifungal cream to apply twice a day and when I apply it to my fingers they bleed. I may stop using the medication. No one really knows what to do with this condition which started in late December other than wait and see.

Helping others - 2/22/11

Have you ever wondered why the title of my home page is The Chosen One? A few months prior to my diagnoses I woke up from a dream where I was in a room and a voice said, "You are the Chosen One". At the time, I was contemplating writing a book and thought well maybe that should be the title of my book. Now, I realize that it meant so much more. I am adamant about helping others as I continue to move through this journey. On Sunday, I attended my first support group meeting with the local Central VA chapter of the Sister Network. By joining this national organization, I will be able to reach out to a larger audience in helping others in need. I'm excited and blessed to walk into this ministry.

Bouncing back - 3/1/2011

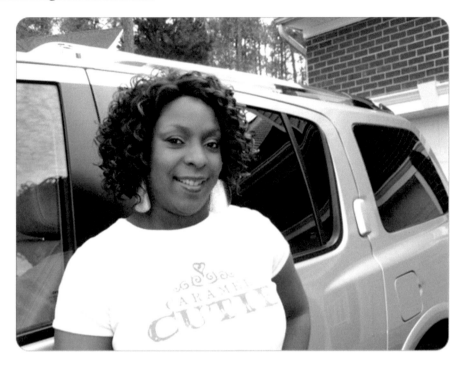

It's time to bounce back from the effects of all the chemo drugs & radiation. My energy level is beginning to increase. I have returned to belly dancing and took my first Zumba class. My flexibility is not where it was but I'm on my way. Also, neuropathy has my balance off at times. My fingers are not bleeding as frequently so I'm prayerful that they are beginning to heal.

Continuing to heal - 3/8/2011

My strength and energy level are slowly but surely returning. I've been exercising to rebuild my muscles - Zumba, Belly Dancing, Line Dancing, Wii Let's Dance & Wii Michael Jackson Experience. So much fun!!! Although Michael Jackson's Thriller & Tina Turner's Proud Mary had all of us sore for days. I never realized how good it felt to exercise until it was taken away from me. My fingers continue to provide me with some challenges as well as the numbness in my feet BUT I'm not going to focus on that - I'm going to just keep it moving. Oh yeah, and I've been busy planning my 40th birthday party - Boy, do I have a reason to celebrate!

Treatment day - 3/10/2011

It's Treatment Thursday. I'm getting ready to go for my Herceptin cocktail and then sleep the day away. My energy level continues to increase - I've gone a few days without taking an afternoon nap. I believe exercise has been a big help for regaining myself. I've been keeping myself busy with preparing to return to work on April 1st, planning my 40th birthday party, & most importantly planning my annual trip to Aruba.

Under the age of 40 - 3/14/2011

Over the weekend I attended an incredible forum for African American women diagnosed under the age of 40. It was truly an amazing experience to hear the stories from these remarkable women. I'm eagerly looking forward to meeting more people involved in this new initiative. Also, I have been invited to attend the 12th Annual National African American Breast Cancer Conference in Baton Rouge, LA to share my survivor story. God just keeps on allowing me to be used, I'm so blessed!

Unexpected blessing - 3/16/2011

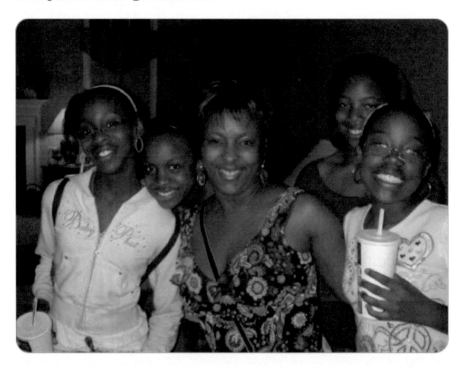

Yesterday, I attended a tour with my daughter for a specialty high school she is considering. The mother of one of her friends asked me to sit by her so she could talk to me. She went on to tell me that she heard from the kids that I had breast cancer and that she was recently diagnosed. She indicated that she was confused and overwhelmed with all of the information. I will be meeting with her soon to help her digest the information so she can make informed decisions. We must all remember to Stop the Silence so that we can be a blessing to others.

God is truly amazing! "You never know when you might be a blessing to others. Always be ready to testify about the greatness of God." ~ Leslie Michelle

Fabulous Forty - 3/22/2011

I just concluded a 72hr birthday party with my family & friends. We all had the time of our life. I wanted to ensure that it was a special event for all - there was a cocktail party, a brunch, a party, & a cookout. It was amazing to see so many people who came from so many places: Boston, Atlanta, Charlotte, Charleston, Columbia, Washington DC, & Norfolk. I'm truly blessed and thankful to be alive with so many wonderful people in my life.

Helping others - 3/24/2011

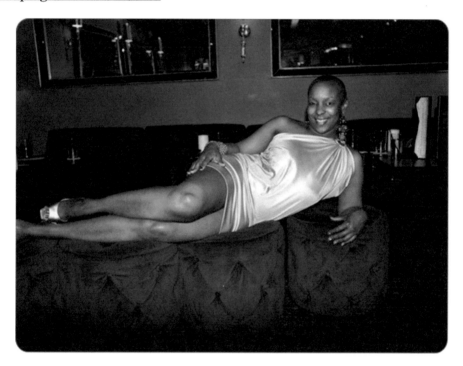

Today I find myself thanking God for allowing me to be here to help my sisters who are coming behind me. Today, I have a friend who begins chemo & another who is getting her port installed. Almost daily, I'm assisting someone with understanding their diagnosis or treatment options. Wow - is this not crazy! This disease is running rampant, and we are all clueless to why.

"Sisters, we must keep on fighting the fight. Keep yourself surrounded by positive people and positive energy. At all times be a light to help illuminate the path of those who may be following you - often we do not even know that they are in our shadows." ~Leslie Michelle

Healthy Heart - 3/28/2011

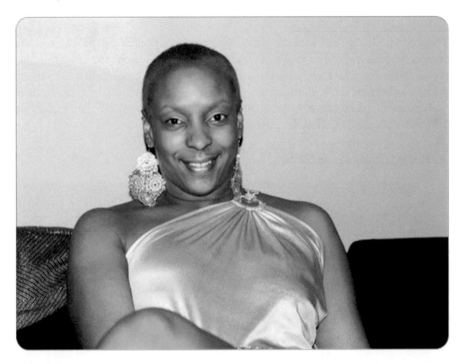

Today I went to see a cardiologist. The doctors have been running test and watching me closely because I did not feel well after my last Herceptin treatment on March 10th. It appears that the asthmatic symptoms may have been related to my seasonal allergies. Everything looks ok with my heart. Thank God for small miracles - next treatment is this Thursday. Have I told you how wonderful it feels to be 40yrs old? I'm having the time of my life.

Treatment Day - 3/31/2011

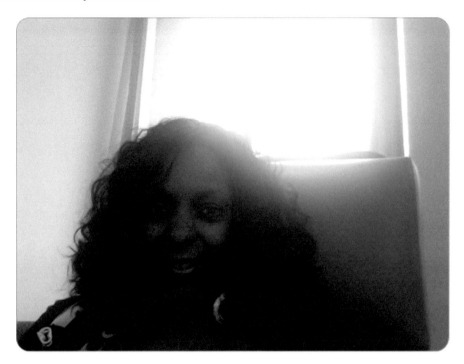

Look at what I picked up at the treatment center today. A cute black lace front wig. Think I will wear it to my belly dance performance. I'm being silly & having fun. Wouldn't it be cool to freak everyone out when I return to work on Monday by wearing a different wig each day? LOL

5 LIFE AFTER TREATMENT

Return to work - 4/4/2011

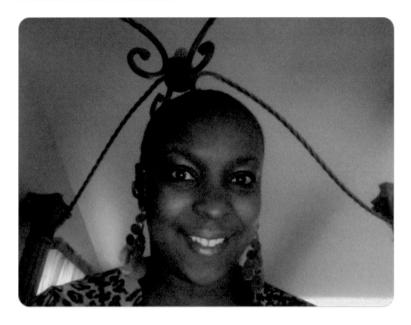

Today, I returned to work. Let's just say that I will need a constant reminder of why I do what I do: I love to travel, I have kids to support, and I like having shelter, food, & clothing. Everything is crazy in the office. New manager, new group, new hires. It is true insanity, and they are ready to dump any and everything on me.

Business as usual - 4/14/2011

So this is my second week back on the job. In typical corporate fashion, I've been thrown on a project that is behind schedule and must be completed by the end of June. Lots of work and not enough time. But rest assured that I'm keeping everything in perspective. I'm working a normal full-time schedule, not staying late, and not working weekends. If it is completed on time great and if it is not that is great too. Going through what I have experienced makes it even easier to maintain a proper work/life balance. My energy level is returning to almost normal. I've been exercising and dancing as I prepare for a performance on Mother's Day weekend. Yes, I've just returned to work and I'm looking forward to my Aruba vacation next month! Have a great day.

Relapse - 4/18/2011

So now that I have worked for two weeks, my problematic finger has started to flare up again. I've been placed back on antibiotics to clear up the infection. Here we go again......

Own your health - 4/21/2011

I'm at the cancer center getting my Herceptin treatment. Feeling a little high from the drugs and looking forward to the wonderful nap that follows. Today I told one of my research nurses to write me a 90-day supply of vitamin D and if today's lab work shows that my level is too low, I will fill the prescription. The nurse wanted to know which doctor ordered the vitamin D work - you should have seen his face when I told him that I ordered it. ROFL - "Just wanted to remind everyone that you are empowered, and you must own your health. Never assume that your medical team has full accountability for your well-being. It must be a partnership - you must contribute." ~Leslie Michelle

Feeling good - 5/9/2011

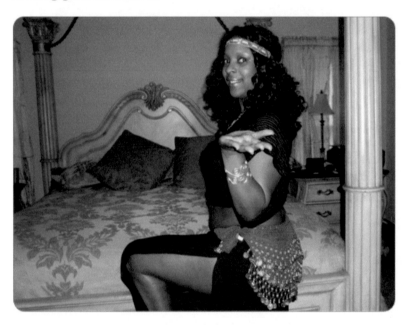

I'm feeling good! Reclaiming my life and doing things I have never done before. Here is one of my alter egos, Sa' Diya as I was preparing for my first Belly Dance performance. It was so much fun. "Enjoy life now. Do whatever your heart desires. Don't worry about what others think - have fun. Rest when you are Dead." ~Leslie Michelle

Dr. Wilson - 5/11/2011

Just call me Dr. Wilson. Upon arriving at the cancer treatment center today, the first thing I did was to request the FSH & LH lab work. My doctor and assigned nurse were not available to give the formal orders so I issued it on their behalf. The chemo nurse will run the test and let them know that I authorized it.

LMAO What is FSH & LH you ask? (FSH = Follicle Stimulating Hormone. LH = Luteinizing Hormone). These are the reproductive or fertility hormones that will show if I'm officially in menopause or not. I'm praying that I'm officially infertile because I sure am enjoying a life without a menstrual cycle.

Survivor's Conference - 5/17/2011
Over the weekend, I attended the 12th National Sister's Network Conference in Baton Rouge, LA. I was the keynote speaker giving my Survivor's story. It was an amazing experience. God allowed me to be used to motivate and inspire hundreds of women. I cannot adequately put into words how rewarding this conference was. There were scientists, physicians, and surgeons who were the best in their fields as presenters. Not only did they provide valuable information but also was able to answer personal questions. I Thank God for affording me this opportunity and for my friends who were able to look out for my children while I was away.

Aruba Time - 5/24/2011

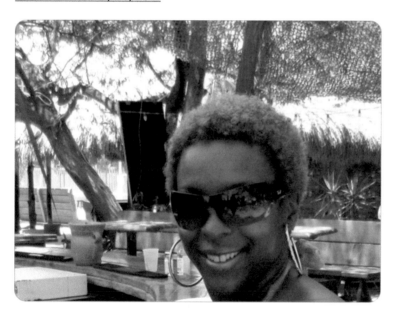

Time to head out for the annual girls' trip to Aruba. I have a 7am light. There are 10 ladies traveling with me this year - can't wait to have fun in the sun. Last time this year I was on top of the world. As soon as I returned from Aruba, I discovered the lump. Wow - it is hard to believe that a year has passed already. "God your wonders still amaze me. Thankful for your grace and favor - recognizing that I don't deserve it but you just keep on blessing me". ~Leslie Michelle

Return from Aruba - 6/1/2011

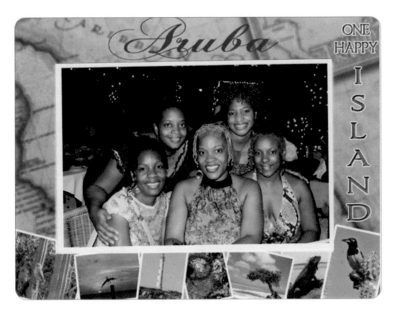

Just returned from my 7th annual trip to Aruba. It was a total of 10 ladies this year and we had a blast. Who said you can't be sexy after breast cancer? Wrong!!! I wore my standard bikini with my port just to prove the point. No one knew unless I told them my story. "Living a full life and enjoying EVERY minute of it". ~Leslie Michelle

It's Official - 6/23/2011

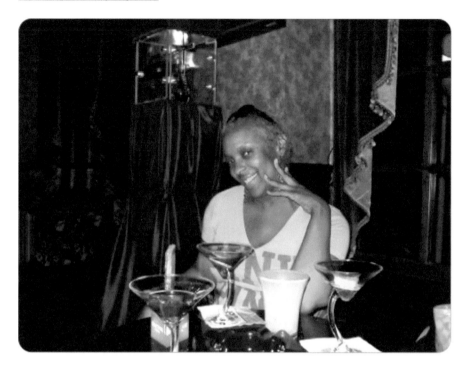

Yesterday I had a check-up and asked my oncology nurse to look at the results of my blood work I ordered about a month ago to determine if I am officially in menopause. The results are that I am postmenopausal - Hip, Hip, Hooray! This is one benefit of chemo that is something to brag about!!! No more monthly visitors at age 40 - yes!

Mixed Emotions - 6/24/2011

I just looked at the calendar and noticed the date - June 24th. For many years this has been a date that represented joyous events such as my parents' anniversary and the birthdate of my aunt, Sheena Wright (RIP). But now there is also an additional item that I have added to my memory bank. On this day 1 year ago, I received the results from my biopsy - "You have breast cancer". So today, I reflect on the last year of my life and the journey that I have been on. I have met some incredible people and have been enjoying those whom I love and cherish.

"Thank You, God, for revealing to me that I had this dreadful disease, for holding me up when I was low, for providing me with friends and family to be my anchor, and for renewing my body and soul." ~Leslie Michelle

Party with a purpose - 6/27/2011

I had a wonderful weekend hanging out with Hiliary, Von, Rhonda, Kim, and Moni. We started with the R Kelly Love Letter Concert in Raleigh and ended it with Steve's annual Birthday Bash in Washington DC. This year Steve's party had a twist. It was an All-White Party with pink accents. There was breast cancer awareness and vendors on site. Part of the proceeds were to support the breast cancer war. It was an amazing, grown, and sexy event!!!

Anniversary - 7/8/2011

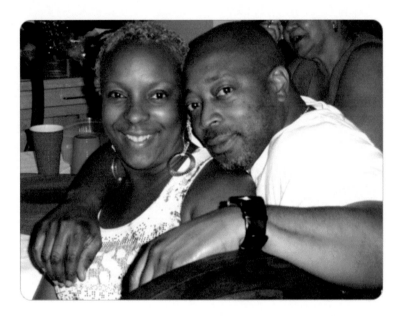

Do you know what today is? It's my anniversary! one year cancer-free
I have 2 more treatments left and I'm enjoying every day to its fullest.

Thanking God for his favor!!!! Thanking God for my family and friends.

~"I love you all more than you will ever know but I pray that my actions will give you an indication of what you mean to me". ~Leslie Michelle

-

Tea Time - 7/10/2011

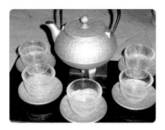

For many years now, I have wanted a tea set. A couple of years ago while vacationing in Mexico I saw a beautiful sterling silver set but did not purchase it. Yesterday, I met friends for tea at Teavana and then brunch. There was this beautiful set that looked like a color between pink and lavender that I just couldn't resist. So tonight, I'm sitting on my sofa enjoying a cup of tea and admiring my authentic Japanese cast iron set. You would think that I just won the lottery - It is amazing how full I get from the simple pleasures of life.

Winding down - 7/14/2011

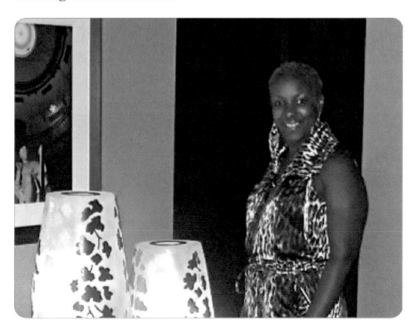

Time is winding down, I'm at the cancer treatment center now. After today, I have one more appointment and then I'm done with this chapter. It is still hard to believe the journey I have been on over the past year. It feels like this has been a very long nightmare and I will wake up soon. My prayer is that this is completely behind me.

Bone Density test - 7/19/2011

Yesterday, I went in for a bone density test known as DEXA. The purpose of this test was to determine if I had chemo-induced osteoporosis. This test was very similar to getting an x-ray. I simply lay on my back fully dressed and a scan of my spine and hips was done. The result was that I have very minimal damage that can be repaired by taking a daily calcium supplement.

Survivorship Plan - 7/26/2011

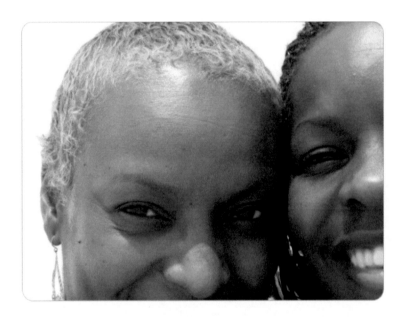

Can you imagine how overwhelming it is for a cancer survivor to keep up with appointments? I am extremely organized, and it is still a lot to manage. But there is great news to share. The medical community is stepping up the game and proactively assisting patients and caregivers. Many hospitals are beginning survivorship clinics with the sole purpose of creating survivorship plans. A Survivorship Plan summarizes your diagnosis, treatment, medication, and side effects into a comprehensive document. This plan allows for effective communication and information sharing between all members of your medical team. It is also a valuable tool if you decide to move and obtain new doctors.

So, now I have added an additional resource to my team. I have a Survivorship nurse and yes, I have a Survivorship plan which outlines every appointment I should have over the next 10 years. Amazing!

Final Herceptin Treatment - 8/4/2011

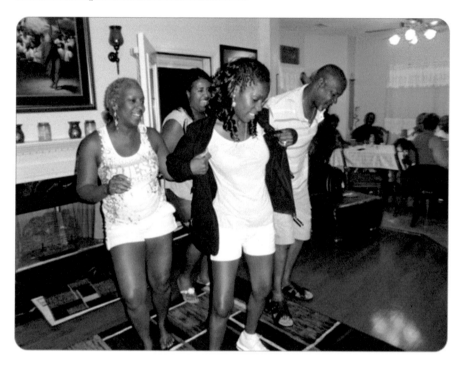

It's party time! Today is my final Herceptin treatment and also I took my last Tykerb pills this morning. I was so excited and eagerly awaiting this day that I could not sleep peacefully last night. I woke up at 5 am this morning and had no problem jumping out of bed. Thankful that this part of the journey is behind me. As Jennifer Hudson said when she won her Oscar, "Look at What God Can Do".

"Look at What God Can Do" - this is what Jennifer Hudson said when she won her Oscar. It touched my hurt because it was genuine and not the standard, "I want to Thank God" rehearsed lines that so many celebrities deliver. So at this moment, all I can say is Look at What God Has Done for Me.- Early Diagnosis- Removed Fake Friends- Elevated Real Friends- Paid my Bills- Saved my Job- Healed my Body "And if God never does anything else for me, I sure as heck can't complain. He has been and continues to be an amazing force in my life." ~ Leslie Michelle

Mammogram - 8/08/2011

I started this morning with my baseline mammogram. It was very painful, which is to be expected after receiving radiation. After the first images, I was asked to come back and take additional pictures of my left breast. Of course, this made me very nervous. After the additional pictures, I was then asked to get dressed and come to Dr. Paredes' office. I was so relieved when she walked in with a big smile on her face. Everything looks good - she just wanted to catch up with me. I will have another mammogram in 6 months as suggested by the National Cancer Association.

Follow-up with Oncologist - 8/11/2011
I had my follow-up appointment today with my Oncologist. My tumor markers look good, and she has given me the ok to schedule my port removal. That is great news; especially since I already have the surgery scheduled for Monday morning. LOL
You know I'm optimistic, proactive, and a planner. All of the appointments that they would have told me to schedule, I have already made. I can't help myself - it's my life and I'm not depending on them to remember EVERYTHING that I need! Life is great - I feel good, I'm exercising, I'm dancing, and I'm eating healthy again! Who could ask for much more?!

Port Free! - 8/15/2011

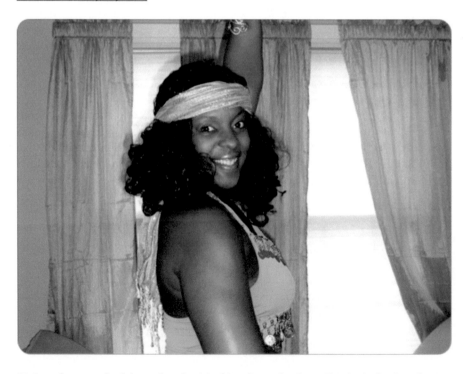

Enjoyed a wonderful weekend with friends at the Jazz Festival. And woke up early today because I was looking forward to my outpatient surgery this morning to remove my port. Thank You Jesus!!!! Woo Hoo!

Echo Today - 8/17/2011

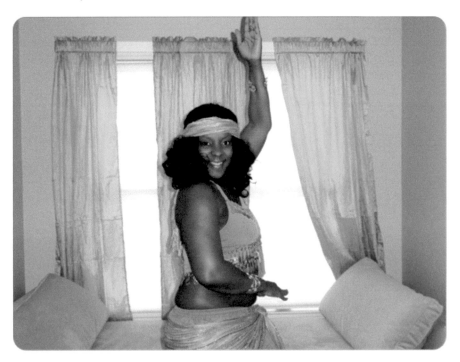

Today, I had my follow-up Echo to make sure there was no damage to my heart from the chemo drugs. I've been pretty sore the last couple of days from the surgery on Monday to remove my port. I've been taking it easy and refraining from exercising this week. I pray that this will heal quickly because my next dance performance is only 10 days away.

I'm Gonna Luv U Through it - 8/18/2011

This debuted on the Today Show this morning and I thought I would share it with all of those who LOVED me through it.
Thank You for being a part of my support system. You kept my spirits up, you took me to the doctor's appointments, cooked my meals, and made me laugh. I LOVE YOU more than you'll ever know. Martina McBride - I'm Gonna Love You Through It https://youtu.be/ZYNOXRifXKQ?si=cxm251hxJl8a97q4

20/20 - 8/30/2011

Great News! I had my eyes checked today and my vision is still 20/20 - Thank God the chemo drugs have not destroyed my vision. But I'm still suffering from chemo brain fog. It is REAL!

MRI Hell! - 9/4/2011

I've had my 2nd unsuccessful attempt at an MRI this month. On the 1st attempt, the technician could not find a vein. On the 2nd attempt, I had an expert who still had trouble but was able to access it via my wrist. The first 20 minutes were fine and then she began the contrast. As soon as the chemical hit my stomach, I got sick all over the table. I was miserable but continued with the procedure. The next day, I received a phone call indicating that there was too much movement during the procedure and that I would have to repeat it for a 3rd time. Very, very frustrating!

Trying something new - 9/21/2011

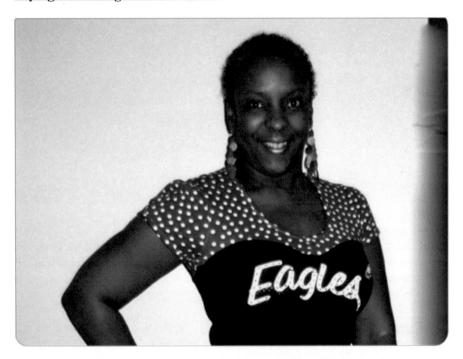

Last week I began swimming lessons for the first time in my entire life. I'm so proud of myself - I learned to put my head underwater, float on my stomach, float on my back, and begin to kick. I hope I'm able to continue with the lessons but with my demanding schedule, it is very difficult. "What have you done this week, this month, or this year that you have never done before"? ~Leslie Michelle

MRI success - 9/21/2011

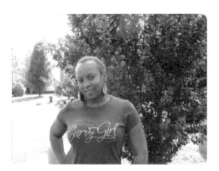

I am happy to report that I was able to have a successful MRI today. The doctor called with the results, and everything was clear. Praise God!

Costume Party 2011 - 10/24/2011

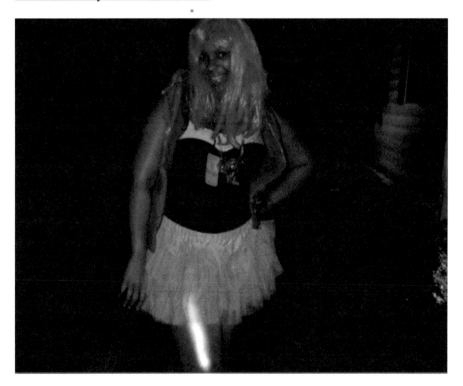

This year's costume for the annual Halloween party was Nicki Minaj. The theme was come as a celebrity with red carpet & pictures in front of a custom step and repeat. Enjoying life!!!!!

Celebrating Survivorship - 10/20/2011

1 in 8 women will be diagnosed with breast cancer. Within the Girls Night Out (GNO) crew 2 of 5 were diagnosed within months of each other. We are survivors- GO GET CHECKED. Talk to your family about your history. Don't be fooled by thinking that YOU won't get it because it doesn't "run" in your family.

Check-up - 11/4/2011

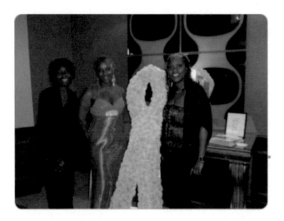

Today was my 3-month checkup with the Oncologist. It was a good day because they were able to draw blood on the first attempt. Because my veins are so small, they have to stick me in my wrist - Ouch! Blood counts have recovered, and I will receive the results of the additional test in a couple of days. In a few hours, I will be headed to Negril, Jamaica with my official GNO (Girls Night Out) crew. So blessed to have my dad drive all the way here just to stay with the kids and give me a break.

Grieving - 11/21/2011

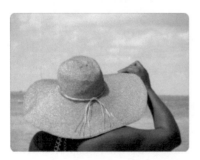

I learned today that a friend passed last Saturday. I thought I should share her story with you again because it may save your life or someone you know. She had what she believed was shingles - a rash on her chest. No lump! No discharge - just a rash. In December, she felt very bad and went to the ER where she was told that she had breast cancer, not shingles. At the time she was diagnosed, it was Stage IV. Over the last couple of months, I was blessed to have gone to lunch with her and share information regarding treatment and options. My prayers go out to her family & I pray that my friend is resting peaceful in the arms of Jesus.

Happy New Year - 1/01/2012

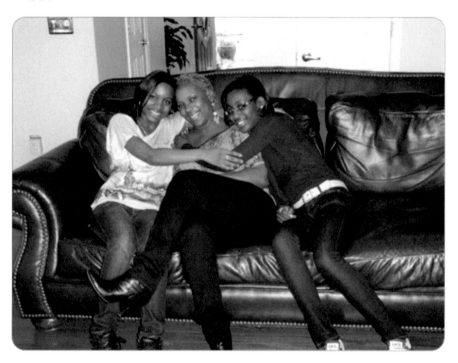

As I reflected over the last year, I'm overwhelmed with emotions. God has brought me so far in such a short period of time. It all seems like a bad dream but the scar that I see every day reminds me of how blessed I am. As I try to make continuous improvements in my life, I've decided to take a break from meat. It has been two weeks now. My body feels wonderful - I have noticed an increase in my energy level. I have also begun juicing. Wishing you all a year of love, happiness, good health & tremendous wealth. Blessings!

Special Days - 2/1/2012

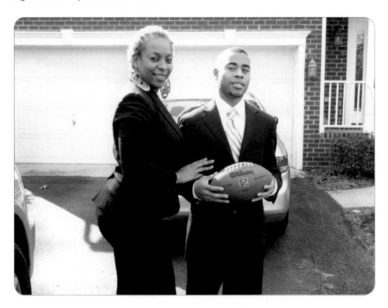

I attended a survivor luncheon a few months back sponsored by the Susan Komen organization. One thought we were left with was, "What I would have missed?" Today, I was blessed to share in my son's happiness at his signing day ceremony for his NCAA football commitment to attend North Carolina Wesleyan College. Thank You, God, for your continued blessings.

Reliving my teen years - **3/7/**2012

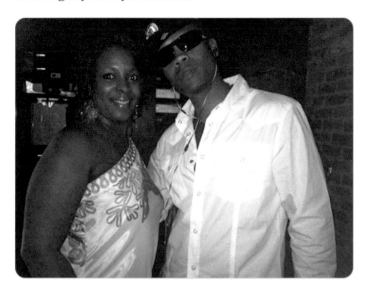

I just completed another check-up, and everything is still looking great. Thank God! I am truly enjoying my life – EVERY DAY. Over the weekend, I was blessed to run into one of my first true loves at a CIAA party. Ronnie DeVoe, member of BBD / New Edition. This was about 30 years overdue. LOL It was great to re-live my teenager years.

Great News - 3/16/2012

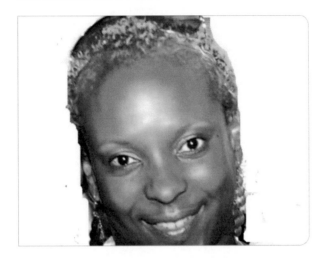

Yesterday, I had my 6month checkup and everything continues to look great. The mammogram was clear! In September, I will have my final mammogram & MRI then return to annual check-ups.

This week, I have spoken to a couple of friends all with scares that proved to be false alarms. This is Great News - I'm so happy that everyone is paying attention to their bodies and taking the appropriate actions. Early Detection Saves Lives!

Remember, continue to be aware of your body not just your breast but all of you.

Happy New Year - 1/2/2013

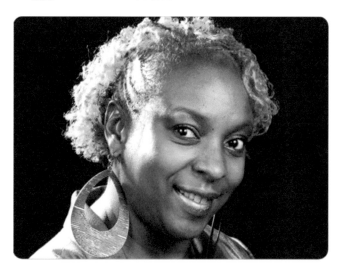

Happy New Year to all. I know it has been a few months since I submitted an entry. Unfortunately, Apple's Mobile Me service discontinued hosting websites so I had to find a new home. I'm in the process of reformatting the website so be on the lookout for changes in the new year. Life continues to be great for me. I have met some incredible survivors who have ventured down this journey after me. Each of them has inspired me to continue the communications that I have started so that our light can continue to shine. Blessings ~Ms Leslie

6 SECOND DIAGNOSIS

Unexpected Visitor - 10/9/2013

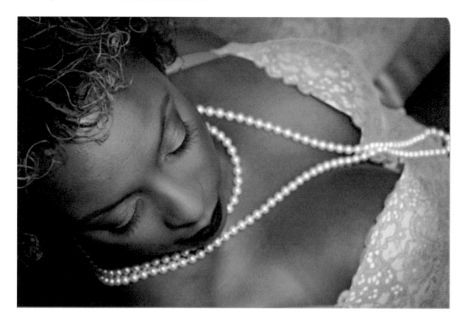

The last couple of months have been crazy. Lots of changes. On Sept. 25th I had my annual mammogram & MRI. The mammogram came back clear, and I got a good bill of health. Then to my surprise, I received a phone call later that same evening telling me that something on the MRI was suspicious. Unfortunately, the biopsy indicated a new cancer in the opposite breast. I have requested a bilateral mastectomy along with reconstruction. Now, I am preparing for the next phase of this journey. Thank you all for the many calls, texts, and prayers. As always, I look at things in a positive light. I get to choose what type of boobies I want to have. I'm going to have some fun with this. Stay tuned.

Surgery Scheduled - 10/10/2013

I received a call yesterday with my surgery date. It is set for Monday, Oct. 28th. I'm expected to remain in the hospital for 2 days and will have approximately 6–8-week recovery. The timing for all of this seems horrible but God is in charge so I'm not going to sweat it. Random Thought: Everyone knows how horrible the economy is so being laid off right now seems like a dead end. It's been a little over a month and I have received 3 exciting job offers plus working on starting a business. Of course, I had to turn all of the job offers down because of my surgery. I'm convinced this is just a sign of God's continued favor over my life. What's for me is mine and it will be there waiting for me when I'm ready.

Preparations Begin - 10/14/2013

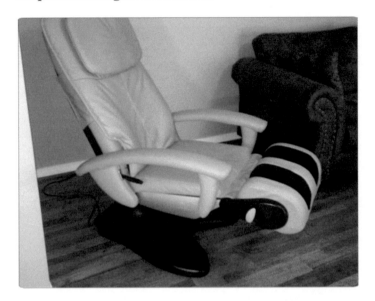

Blessings!!!! Look at this amazing massage chair that a fellow survivor / Komen volunteer GAVE to me. I have begun preparing for my surgery which is approximately 2 weeks away. I ordered a recliner for my bedroom and today went shopping at Sam's to stock up on staple household items. Busy, busy, busy as I prepare to ensure that my household continues to run smoothly while I am recuperating. "Thank You, God for my amazing friends and families. And Lord gives them plenty of strength and patience because they will have to deal with me. Lord, you know I'm not the easiest person to live with. You know all my little pet peeves - the things that drive me crazy cause you created me so help me to ignore those things and appreciate all the love that continues to surround me. Self-awareness is half the battle! " ~Leslie Michelle

Pre-Op Begins - 10/15/2013

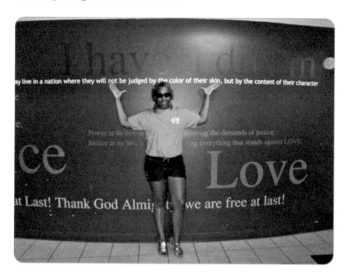

Today was a long day at the hospital. I had a CT scan with contrast and radioactive Bone Scan completed. I've been drinking lots of water to flush the chemicals out of my system. Now the countdown is on...... the time is drawing near for me to get my new "girls". I took this photo when visiting Atlanta in August. "I have a dream that I will be cancer-free for life!"

Feeling Blessed - 10/17/2013

I wish I could explain to you why I still have the joy that I do despite the bumps in the road. All I can say is "But God" - my joy doesn't come from the world. Feeling blessed with all the special people in my life. I'm convinced that my friends are the most amazing on the planet! I received an exciting email today that I can't wait to share the details with you all. But this is Thursday so just like my favorite show Scandal, you are going to have to wait a few days for the surprise. Love You All!

To Reconstruct or Not? - 10/23/2013

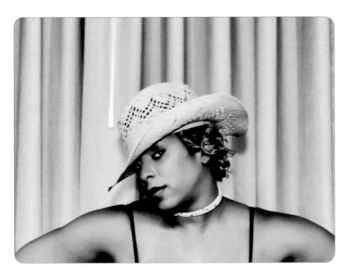

After a couple of weeks of soul-searching, I have made the decision that I will not have reconstruction surgery along with my mastectomy. Instead, I will have a unique tattoo mural designed to cover my chest. Some of you may wonder or not even understand how I could opt to go this route but as you know it is a very personal decision. For me, I have always been against cosmetic enhancements of any type. I have always been comfortable in my skin - flaws and all. The thought of having implants did not sit well with me. The thought of feeling like I am constantly wearing an underwire bra because of the procedure also does not sit well with me. The long-drawn-out procedure and additional surgeries along with the possibility of infections were also deterrents. On Monday of this week, I called and canceled the plastic surgeon. I'm happy to have this decision behind me since it has preoccupied my thoughts, and I am excited about working with the artist to create a unique design.

"Lord, I sure hope that my recovery is speedy 'cause I got some stuff I need to do. Speedy like let's be over this in about 2 weeks. I need to get my business off the ground and you know Thanksgiving is coming and I have to make my goodies. Especially the sweet potato blueberry pies." ~Leslie Michelle

<u>Acts of Kindness - 10/25/2013</u>

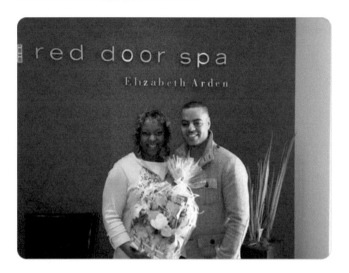

My family and friends all know that I am a "Giver". I thrive on doing for others and often find it difficult to sit back and simply receive Acts of Kindness. Today was an exception to the rule. I was treated to a spa treatment at one of my favorite places, Red Door Spa. Upon checking out of the spa, I was informed that I had visitors, A Top-Notch marketing executive, and supporting staff. (I thought there was a change in their schedule, and I would not be able to meet them as previously planned). Not only was I able to personally thank the marketing team who arranged the spa day but to my surprise John Michael was waiting in the lobby. I was serenaded by John Michael who performed his song, Sophisticated Lady. Everyone knows how much I love music so this was a special treat & the brother can SING!!!! I was blown away. Red Door Spa & Top-Notch Marketing, thank you for supporting the cause. Central VA Komen Foundation, I am so happy to be a part of this family and humbled by all of the love you have shown. John Michael, only a special person takes time out of their schedule to visit a stranger in another city simply to say, "You are Appreciated". "When I think about all of the special people that have come into my life through this journey, all I can say is Thank You Jesus for continuing to shower me with blessings.

"At all times continue to praise him. Remain optimistic. Don't let anyone or anything steal your joy!" ~Leslie Michelle

The Big Day is Tomorrow - 10/27/2013

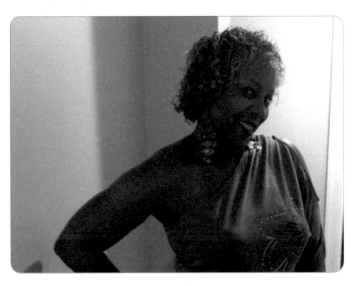

Today, I enjoyed a wonderful service and church and received encouragement from all of my "church neighbors" (the folks who sit near me each Sunday). The Big Day is tomorrow. My surgery is at 7:30 am and is expected to last approximately 2 hrs. Mom & Dad have arrived and will be staying with me to assist for a few weeks. My daughter and friends have reminded me that they are expecting me to be back to baking peach cobbler and sweet potato blueberry pies within 2-3 weeks. They don't care how it happens as long as I make it happen :) So I'm sure you are wondering, how am I really feeling inside? I am feeling a little anxious. Nervous about anesthesia and wondering what challenges I will face learning to accept my new body. Will I be completely shocked at my new figure? Will I have challenges figuring out how to dress for a new body? Will I have to completely replace my wardrobe? These are a few of the thoughts that are going through my head. Despite all these thoughts running through my head, I'm still smiling and full of joy both inside and out. Crazy I know but the only way I can explain it is to encourage you to get in a personal relationship with God and see what he will do for you. The peace he places over your soul is indescribable. Now I will prepare all my notes for my helpers and finish packing my bag for my hospital stay. (Silk bonnet, silk pajamas, iPod so I can jam in the operating room, what else do I need to pack?) Love You All - Thanks for the prayers, cards, and treats. Talk to you soon!

7 MASTECTOMY

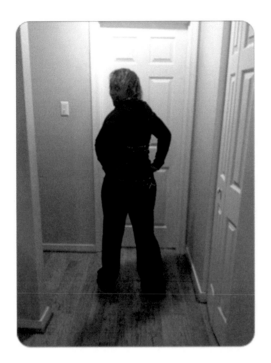

Mastectomy Day Arrives - 10/28/2013

I have many special songs. One of them that I often listen to on my drive to church is "Can't Give Up Now"- by Mary Mary, "There will be mountains that I will have to climb And there will be battles that I will have to fight. But victory or defeat, it's up to me to decide. But how can I expect to win If I never try". And you all know that I rarely back down from a fight! Thanking God for my strength that I know comes from him and him alone. PS I hope you can see the writing on my sweats. It says, "Breast Cancer can Kiss my Butt!" - Love YA! Muah :> On my way now.

Surgery is Over - 10/28/2013

Just wanted everyone to know that I am doing well. In case you are wondering why I look so cozy, it's because I convinced them to release me from the hospital. That's right - I'm back home. More importantly, I am feeling really good about the decision I made. Surrounded by family & friends feeling blessed! Jill Scott - Blessed I woke up in the morning feeling fresh to death I'm so blessed, yes yes I went to sleep stressed, woke up refreshed I'm so blessed, yeah yes Water in my face and everything is in its place Peace of mind even my grace I'm so blessed, yes yes yes That about sums it up for me. I'm going to take it easy, so I don't have any complications. Peace & Blessings!!!!

Friends & Family! - 10/29/2013

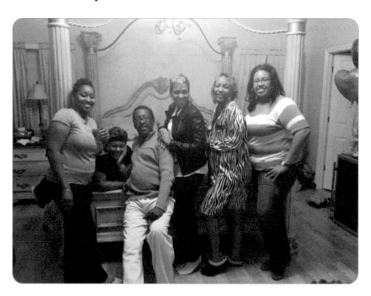

I know many of you planned to stop by the hospital to check on me but you will have to detour to my home instead. :) Surprised everyone by treating this surgery as an outpatient procedure. That's right surgery at 7:30am and headed home at 2pm. Look at what God can do!!!! So, Thank You All because I'm sure your prayers had a lot to do with my strength. Who would ever think that a person could say, "I had a great Mastectomy Day" but I did. As you can tell by the picture above taken in my bedroom with a few of my friends who dropped by. Love this crazy crew & the party we had last night!!!!

No More Meds - 10/31/2013

Recovery is in full effect. Today, I have gone cold turkey - no more pain medication. The best way to describe how I am feeling is a car accident. The muscles in my back are incredibly sore and I have some swelling under my left arm where a few lymph nodes were removed. Overall, I'm impressed at how well I am doing. Especially since sitting still drives me absolutely crazy! Mom & Dad have me locked down. The warden "Mom" is making sure I don't do anything I am not supposed to do. My parents are so funny; I was laughing so hard today that I thought I was going to bust a stitch. LOL

Praise Report - 11/4/2013

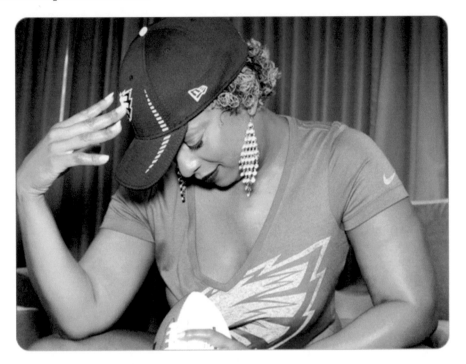

No more drains - Woo Hoo!!!! Today I met with my nurse. She has named me her "Poster Child for Super Woman". She could not believe I checked out of the hospital the same day as my surgery and that I was not on any pain meds. The best part of the visit was receiving my full pathology report which showed there was absolutely no sign of cancer in my body including my breast and lymph nodes. What does this mean? The biopsy that I had on Sept. 30th removed the small cancer tumor completely. The mastectomy that I elected to have was a preventive procedure to help minimize the risk of reoccurrence. What's next? Continue the healing process and meet with my Oncologist on Nov. 19th to find out if any additional medications or chemo is recommended. Thank You Jesus for continuing to Bless Me!!!!

Slow and Steady - 11/11/2013

It's been 2 weeks since my surgery and each day I'm feeling stronger. Today was the first day I drove a short distance because I have limited range of motion with my arms. The next step for me will be physical therapy. I'm dreading the activity but know that it will be instrumental in my healing. "Thank God for mothers. My Mom has been my rock assisting me with all of my needs as I recuperate. ~Leslie Michelle

Guess who can drive again? - 11/16/2013

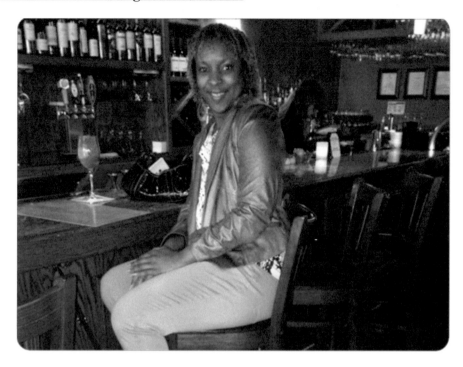

Progress continues through this incredibly humbling experience. Having a limited range of motion with my arms has forced me to rely on others to assist around the house as well as simple tasks like putting on a jacket. My parents were here to assist me, and Mom will be returning to Charleston today, so the real challenge begins. Although many don't believe me, I am truly taking it easy. My easy may not equate to your easy but I am sitting "almost" still. SN: Last night at church I heard a powerful sermon from Pastor E. Dewey Smith from Atlanta on the power of prayer and how it can cause God to shift his plans. Check it out for yourself Exodus 32:9-14. Be Blessed!

Reflecting on Stereotypes - 11/19/2013

Today I woke up reflecting on all of the stereotypes that are often unspoken. In 2010, while going through chemo there were times when I felt strong enough to go to church, but I didn't. I could not risk all of the germs from shaking hands. Likewise, now as I am recovering, I am faced with a similar challenge. Often there are others who make assumptions if a person does not shake their hand or if the handshake is not firm.

"We live in a culture where we are taught certain things that we become conditioned to believe are truths. I challenge you to think about some of the things that you make assumptions about. If a person doesn't shake your hand, perhaps it is because they have an immune system that is compromised. If a handshake is not firm/strong, perhaps it is because they are recovering from surgery and this motion is painful. Realize that everything is not about you!" ~ Leslie Michelle.

8 PREPARING FOR CHEMO ROUND 2

Triple Negative Breast Cancer - 11/20/2013

Yesterday I met with my oncologist to discuss my pathology
report and profile. The great news - there are no signs of cancer in my body all
is clear from the CT Scan, Bone Scan, & Mastectomy. Also, all lymph nodes
were clear as well. The type of breast cancer that was removed is known as
Triple Negative Breast Cancer. What this means is that this cancer is not
affected by hormone treatment so I will not be on any additional pills. My
doctor has suggested that I take 4 doses of chemo drug treatment referred to
as Taxotere Cytoxan because these drugs will reduce my risk of having a
reoccurrence to another part of my body by 22%. I told her that I would think
about it and let her know within the next few weeks. Some of you have asked
how you can have a reoccurrence if you decide to proactively have a
mastectomy. Breast cancer can show up in other areas such as the brain, lungs,
liver, or bones through your bloodstream. Chemotherapy treatment is aimed at
reducing the risk of this type of reoccurrence. "God knew that this day would
come long before I did. He knows the resolution as well. My prayer is that he
reveals to me the course of action that is best for me. Order my steps and I will
follow."

It's Not About Me - 11/21/2013

Over the past few days, I have been in deep thought regarding my next steps. I
have withdrawn from answering questions and emails and have gone into my
prayer closet. As I listened to a sermon from Joyce Meyers this morning my
next steps became clear to me. I have reluctantly decided that I will have the
chemo treatment as a preventative treatment. Why? Because today it was
revealed that my decision although a personal one is NOT about me. Instead,
it is about all of those whose lives I have touched or will touch in the future. It
is about me allowing my light, my strength, and wisdom which flows from God
to be a ray of hope for someone else. Friends & Family Thank You for being
patient as you have dealt with my sometimes abrupt and direct tone. Being in
the "spotlight" does not provide one with the opportunity to process their
thoughts so there are times when I have to shut everything off. "There are some
things I cannot ignore, and my faith is one of them.

"God, I THANK YOU for your favor, your mercy, and the blessings that you
have provided to me. I thank you for CHOOSING me and I pray that I can
make you proud." ~Leslie Michelle

2nd Opinion Scheduled - 11/22/2013

My days have been extremely busy with talking to physicians, dealing with
Cobra insurance, attempting to get on the Affordable Health Care website,
looking for a job, and taking care of my household duties. With all that is going
on the easiest way for me to attempt to keep all informed is to continue to blog
daily. I don't have the bandwidth or energy to tell the same story over and over

again so please understand if I refer you to this site. I'm exhausted :) I have scheduled a consultation at Cancer Centers of America where I will travel to meet with staff for a second opinion regarding my treatment. This will allow me to take a holistic approach (mind, body, & soul) and determine the best course of action. In parallel, I am still waiting for the date for my surgery to have my port installed and begin chemo. My best guess at this time is that it will be around Dec. 15th. Thanks for your continued prayers & support!!!

Headed to Philly - 11/26/2013

Did you see the Philly Eagles play today? Those boys were bad!!! Tomorrow I will be flying to Philly and will begin my consultation (2nd opinion) at the Cancer Treatment Center of America on Tuesday. I am eager and excited to learn what this medical team may have to offer. Here is a high-level summary of what is going on: 1. Consult in Philly 2. Port install & chemo (tentatively scheduled week of Dec. 9th) Some have asked why I am considering chemo. Even though my scans are all clear, chemo is often taken as a preventative treatment to minimize the risk of reoccurrence to another area of the body. Today has been a rough day for my family as it looks as though we may be losing a family member. But we must always remember to Praise God in all things. It is a blessing that he (Uncle Eric) was able to be in his right mind, to confess his sins as well as his love, to listen to Al Green once again, and then to tell everyone he is tired and will be leaving tonight. Only God knows the time.

"This thing we call life is a journey; it is simply a ride. A ride with ups and downs and downs and ups. A ride with detours and alternate routes. As much as we enjoy the ride there comes a time when we must get off. Prayerfully when that time comes, you have found your way to the correct road which will lead you to everlasting life. Do right by people always! Live a life of integrity, honesty, loyalty, and love despite what is going on around you. And never forget that God is your Everything and what you do for him is the ONLY thing that matters". ~ Leslie Michelle

9 TREATMENT CENTER

The CTCA experience - 12/11/2013

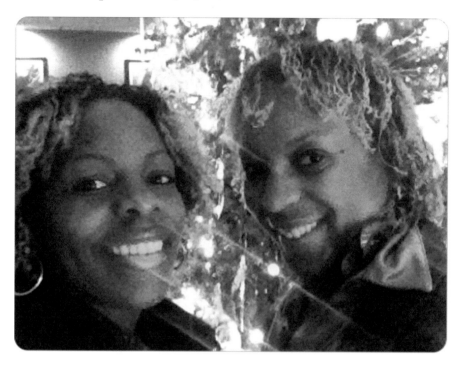

Hello, it's been over a week since I have posted because I did not take my laptop with me to Philly. I have so much to catch you up on. I was at the Cancer Treatment Centers of America, Philadelphia last week. It began with a 3-day consultation followed by a MUGA scan on the fourth day. I was very impressed with the holistic approach and working with a full medical team under one umbrella. The experience at CTCA is amazing. From the doctors, transportation staff, hotel workers, and patients are all unbelievable. It's one big family with a focus on hope, healing, and nothing but positive energy. I was happy to have my sister with me on the tour as well as my ride-or-die friend who made a surprise appearance on the last day. The consult ended with me agreeing to get my treatment at the center and canceling my appointments previously scheduled in Virginia. The treatment I will have is 4 rounds of chemo drug called Adriamycin Cytoxan aka the red devil. Treatments will occur once every 3 weeks. BTW - Last Friday, I flew directly from Philly to Charleston for the Celebration of Life of my favorite uncle, James Eric Wilson. Although we are always sad to see our loved ones go I was happy that his soul was at peace, he said his goodbyes, and that I was able to speak with him before his transition via Skype. RIP Uncle Eric.

Port install & Chemo #1 - 12/11/2013

My Mom flew with me to Philly on Monday and Tuesday, I began round #2 of this cancer journey. The morning began with me having twilight anesthesia (Michael Jackson drugs) to have my port installed followed by my 1st chemo treatment. No issues and the surgeon did an amazing job of putting the port into the same location used previously. Today, I returned to the center where we had a wonderful breakfast, I got my Neulasta shot, and then both Mom & I had our first Reiki massage. It was a cool experience. We took an afternoon flight back to Richmond and now I am home resting with my mom here to assist me.

My New Look - 12/12/2013

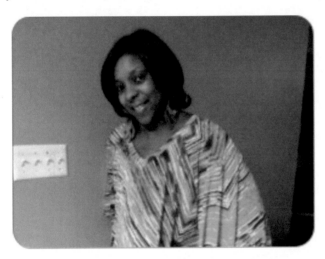

It's so cold this winter (especially in Philly) so I decided to buy a wig this time around. Rather than going to my trusted stylist, I went to a salon that specializes in cancer patients. I allowed the consultant to cut my locks off and shave my hair. I figured I didn't have anything to lose because I would be completely bald in about 10 days. Boy was I wrong, this lady has plugged holes all over my head. LOL - So now, I have no choice but to wear this wig until I am completely bald.

I'm feeling pretty good but have been sleeping most of the day. Not able to eat much and the tiredness is setting in. Thankful that my mom is here to assist me. She is a blessing!

Mctal mouth - Yuck! - 12/13/2013

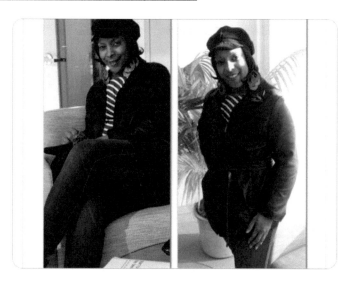

My Mom took these photos of me today. Notice, the silly infamous face on the left that I'm known for making. Now that it is 3 days since my chemo treatment, some of the things that I am experiencing are the nasty metallic taste in my mouth, headaches, sore body (like the flu), and tiredness. Also, having strange food cravings just like pregnancy cravings - for lunch today (all within 5 minutes) I wanted sushi, a steak, corn beef hash, and banana popsicles. I ended up eating the steak and it did not have much of a taste to me but at least I was able to eat today. My body is also craving a lot of sodium (salty plain potato chips) seems to somehow balance the metal taste. Thank God for a good day. Despite having no job, going through chemo, and lots of medical bills, God continues to provide. Still feeling blessed!

Arm Pain - 12/15/2013

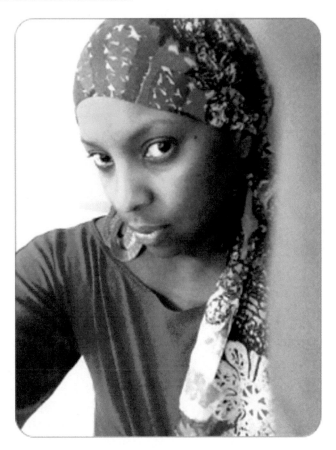

My left arm has been sore and aching since my surgery on Oct. 28th. I can only raise my arm to head level. I'm trying to keep it elevated, but nothing appears to be helping. I thought it would start to feel better by now but instead, it feels worse. I think it may have been aggravated when they strapped my arms down during my surgery last week to install my port. This sucks!!!! Hopefully, I will get some relief when I start physical therapy on Wednesday.

Thought I would have a little fun with a head scarf. This is my Wilona or Chip Fields (Good Times) look. LOL

Axillary web syndrome - 12/19/2013

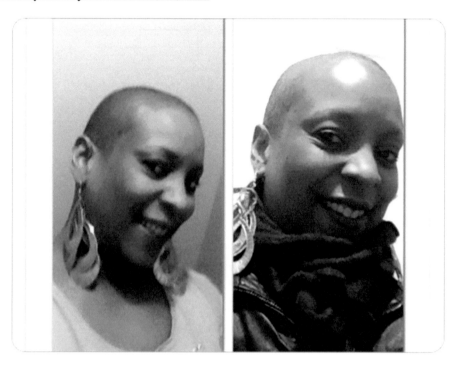

Yesterday, I started physical therapy to regain the full motion of my arms. I knew my left arm was pretty jacked up but didn't realize how bad. So now I have a name for the pain that has been nagging me since my surgery in October. Axillary web syndrome, also referred to as Cording is a condition in which the connective tissues that encase blood vessels, lymph vessels, and nerves become inflamed. For me, this has resulted in a major impact on my daily habits because of the arm pain. Simple things such as reaching over my head and using an ATM or impossible with my left arm. It feels as though you are ripping a muscle apart. In addition to the nasty cording, I woke to severe muscle spasm yesterday in my back. After dealing with it all day, I ended up in an urgent care center last night where I was given some strong drugs and muscle relaxers. What a day!!!! But guess what? I'm still smiling :)

Christmas 2013 - 12/25/2013

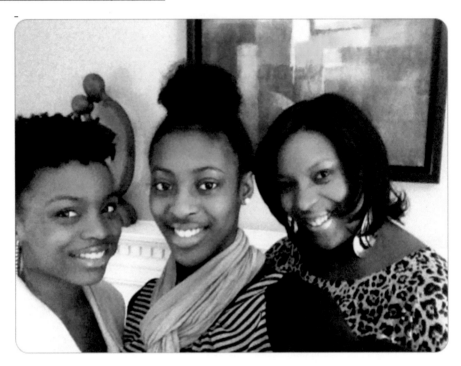

For the first time EVER, the girls and I have spent Christmas away from our family. Although it was not the ideal Christmas, it was still a great day. Great because I know so many people personally who this year are not here to celebrate Christmas. Thanking God for life!

We spent the day with our Richmond family and of course, we ate more than we should have. I cooked a few of our family favorites too - Granny's pineapple cake, chewies, sweet potato blueberry pie, bacon-wrapped shrimp, crab dip, sausage rice, and roasted green beans. It was all delicious!!!!

Hope you all had a Merry Christmas ~ spread love every day!

Better Days - 12/27/2013

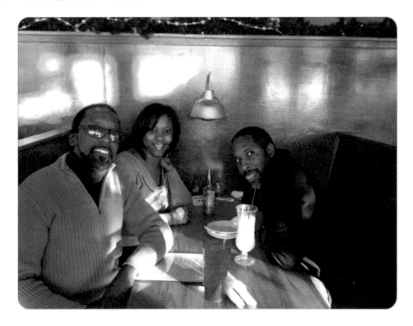

Today I learned what PT stands for and it's not Physical Therapy. PT stands for Pain & Torture but through it all, I was able to extend my arm for the first time in 2 months. So, despite the extreme pain, I was very excited to learn that I may regain the motion in my arm. Chemo#2 Complete - 12/31/2013 First let me start by expressing my joy with the Eagles' victory over the Cowboys, woo hoo! I just returned from Philly today after completing Chemo#2 yesterday and getting my Neulasta shot today. I'm feeling ok - tired & nauseated. It's hard to eat much although I know it is important. I'm trying to get fluids down. On each trip to the Cancer Center, I met some truly amazing survivors and caregivers. That place is truly one of a kind. Well, I'm in bed and not sure that I will be awake to see 2014 roll in so wishing you all a Happy New Year!

Blah - Chemo Nausea - 1/2/2014

Feeling Blah! Chemo Nausea blues - not able to eat or drink much. Thanks to those who have helped me through this round. Due to the complications in my arm and side effects of chemo, I must bring in a housekeeper now to assist me with a few things. She will come once every other week. Not an expense I need to incur right now but I need help. Man down! I'm going to try to eat some soup today. Hope I can get more fluids in to flush my system. Special shout out to my brother from another mother, Marlon, for delivering the peppermint tea, ginger root, & Sugar Shack donut.

Chemo#3 Complete - 1/23/2014

Just returned from Philly where I completed Chemo#3. Because of the winter blizzard that is paralyzing the East Coast, my flight was canceled, and I took a train back home. Last night the body aches began and today I am dealing with the flu-like symptoms. I am 75% complete. One treatment left. Woo Hoo! How am I feeling? I'm feeling great because I am ALIVE. Neuropathy has kicked in, chemo brain on full effect, bouts of insomnia, sore body, and cording still unresolved.

Getting Antsy! - 1/28/2014

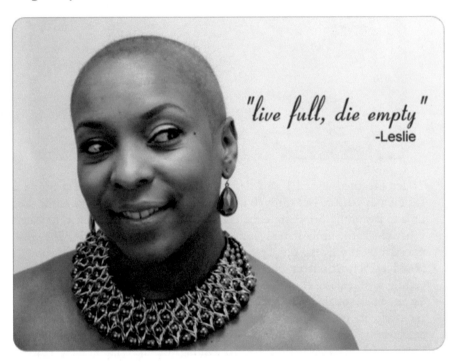

"live full, die empty"
-Leslie

Everyone knows how challenged I am in the "patience" department. This slow recovery is driving me insane. I'm ready to run at full speed without these training wheels on. But instead, I'm trying to take it easy - nausea, hunger, everything is disgusting, metal mouth, and pain in my arm. Cancer Sucks!!!! I decided to take a few professional photos for my business and the photographer threw in a few extras. I believe in the power of positivity. What I mean is this - on the days you see me looking my best it is very likely that I woke up feeling my worst. Put on a cute outfit, cute shoes, makeup, & a smile then your insides will have no choice but to join the party. It's not the easiest thing to do but it sure is worth it. Give it a try!

Chemo is complete! - 2/14/2014

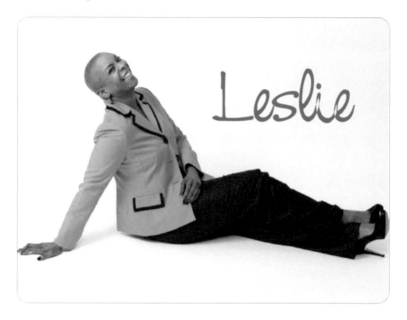

Thank You, Jesus! Chemo is now complete. Next for me is focusing on therapy because I still have very little range of motion with my left arm. I have been in the house all week dealing with the aftermath of the chemo drugs - nausea and fatigue. With all the snow, I did not want to deal with the risk of falling and injuring myself further. Today I celebrate - going to the Maxwell concert tonight. I can't wait!

Let it Flow! - 2/28/2014

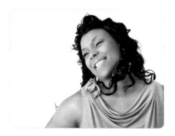

Let it Flow! Your positive energy that is... No matter what is going on, you have a choice on how you will allow it to affect you. I choose to be happy through the ups and downs. What's New? I went to see my surgeon this week and received a referral to a new physical therapist to assist with my axillary cording issues. Got to get this body in shape so I will start next week. Oh yeah, now is the time to return to healthy eating and exercising too. Lots of work today but I'm up for the fight.

10 AFTER CHEMO ROUND 2

Gift from God - 8/17/2014

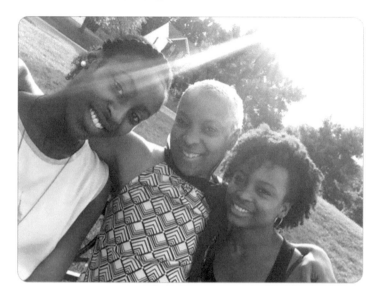

It has been a few months since I have posted. I have been simply enjoying my life including time with my daughters. My oldest is now beginning her first year of college. Woo Hoo!

His Light Within - 9/17/2014

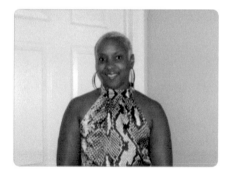

Over the past week, I have come across many angels. Most of them were completely unaware that they were ministering to me. The funny thing is they all felt like I was giving them something but really, they were all giving me so much more. I believe that I am where I am supposed to be. I have a few amazing friends who are all special to me in different ways. I have 2 amazing daughters, I am ALIVE, I am happy, & I am optimistic about what the future holds. My prayer is that I can continue to be a witness to the greatness of God, allowing his Light to shine through me.

<u>Celebrating Life - 9/23/2014</u>

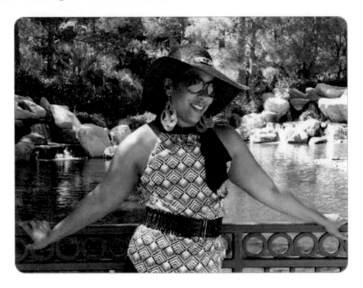

Just returned from the Las Vegas Jazz Festival with one of my girls, Queen. We had an amazing time. The lineup was incredible - it was heaven on earth for true music lovers. We met a few of the performers (which is something I typically do not engage in). I must say that my favorite was Mr. Anthony Hamilton. It was refreshing to see an artist as talented as he is still grounded. My only regret is that his show was cut short - I didn't get to hear my song "Pray for Me" guess that means I will have to catch another show soon :) Feeling like I'm on top of the world! Loving me and loving life.

Happiness is a Choice - 9/24/2014

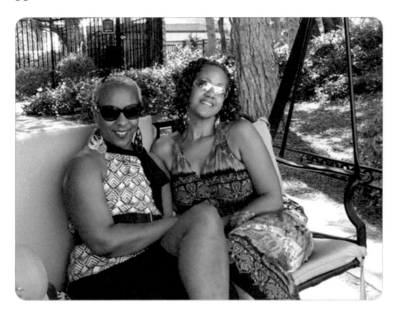

This picture was taken with one of my girls, Queen who joined me for my Vegas Getaway last weekend. A friend in need reached out to me this morning for assistance. She mentioned that she could tell that everything with me must be going well because I look like I'm having fun. I shared with her that Happiness is a Choice. I choose to be happy regardless of the "stuff" that happens to me. I thank God for once again allowing me to minister to someone's soul.

Choose to be Happy. Choose to live in peace & harmony. Choose to surround yourself with positivity and eliminate all things that subtract from you. ~Leslie Michelle

Awareness Month - 10/1/2014

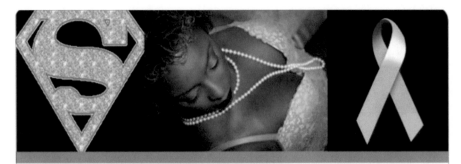

MODERN DAY SHERO

A woman who fights with her mind by believing in supernatural power, having extraordinary faith, maintaining a positive attitude, exuding a loving spirit and still inspiring others through her journey!

10/2/13 Hello Ladies, During my annual MRI a small spot was found in the other breast (7mm in size). This was so small that it was not detected by the new special 3D mammogram that I paid $60 for but it did show on the MRI. Yesterday it was confirmed that it is actually a cancer. So now I am beginning battle#2. I meet with my surgeon tomorrow to discuss my biopsy results and treatment plan. I will be requesting a bilateral mastectomy because I have too much shit to do & cancer is not on my list. Guess this means I will need to have new boudoir photos when I get my new set of DD's since the pair I have now will be replaced Thanks for your willingness to support the cause! Remember to perform your monthly self exams & keep up with your mammograms.

Ladies I can tell you Ellen Parades Imaging Center is the best! People travel from other states to have her and her staff read their charts. My initial diagnosis I discovered myself through a self exam at age 39. No one is immune - at the time I ate healthy, exercised frequently, organic food whole grains, etc. So it can definitely be a shock when you feel that you do all the right things. I refuse to let this disease steal my spirit, drive, or motivation. I got laid off the end of August and preparing to start my business. So I will tell the surgeon let's take them off so I can get this out of my way and on to my big plans.

I am so happy to hear that you ladies are going to get checked.... This is why I have always shared my story. Here is the blog where I tracked my daily journey the first time around. If you go to the Blog page and select go to archives at the bottom of the page, you can see the details from the 1st battle. http://urpowerwithin.com/Welcome.html

10/3/13 I met with my surgeon and I told her that I decided to go with the bilateral mastectomy. Surgery should be in the next 2 - 3 weeks. Next step is to have a consult with a plastic surgeon regarding reconstruction option. At this time I'm on the fence between reconstruction with expanders or simply having a tattoo done across the chest area. My consult with the plastic surgeon is next Tuesday. I know some of you do not know me as well as others but I refuse to be any way except positive. I don't allow negative people in my circle - EVER. With that being said, I'm feeling really blessed today that God has surrounded me with an amazing medical staff. I still have a peace around me that makes no sense at all except to those who are believers. Thanks for your support. I really appreciate the encouraging words you have shared. So in summary, I will have new perky boobies or a HOT ass tattoo. Either way I'm going to be sexy as Hell.

Thankful for all that God has brought me through. Thankful for my voice and my spirit. Prayerful that I am doing what is pleasing to him. Recognizing that a testimony must be shared.

Lean on God - 10/6/2014

I've been in a real funk the last 2 weeks and not completely sure why. I know it doesn't show on my face but it is definitely in my soul. So thankful for true friends - those who I am able to share my most intimate feelings with. And continuing to Lean on God.

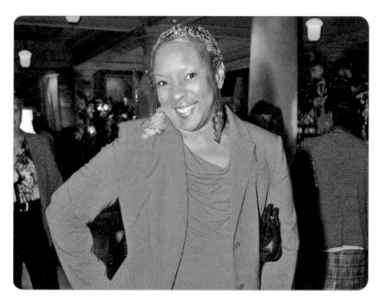

1st Anniversary - 10/28/2014

Wow - Today is the1st anniversary of my surgery. In some ways it is hard to believe that an entire year has passed by. I Thank God for my life! I'm getting stronger and continuing to enjoy every moment. Over this year, I have met some incredible people from many places. I have traveled and spent time enjoying my friendships. I've laughed, I've danced, I've cried, I've prayed, but most of all I have lived!

11 CONCLUSION

As I reflect on my journey, what I want you to know is my life is great! It has been 15 years since my initial breast cancer diagnosis, and I'm still here traveling the world! I share my testimony and encourage others who are embarking on their cancer journey.

I'm often asked if there is anything I would have changed. It's hard to say because looking in the rearview window is always easier. What I can tell you is that while I was going through treatment, my focus was on living, and there wasn't a lot of thought to what life would be like when treatment was over. Perhaps, I would have opted not to endure radiation treatment, bypassed the lumpectomy, and gone straight for the mastectomy.

What I can tell you is that I would not have changed my faith and my commitment to enjoying life every step of the way.

Remember:
1. There is no right or wrong course of treatment, it is a personal decision that only you can make.
2. Guard your peace and block out all negative energy.
3. Live each day authentically!

If you feel like you have questions to ask or simply want to know more, this is just the beginning. It is not the end.

QUESTIONS TO ASK THE SURGEON

1. What type of surgery do you recommend, lumpectomy or mastectomy?
2. What is the estimated stage of my cancer?
3. What type of breast cancer do I have?
4. What are my treatment options?
5. Are there any immunotherapy options instead of chemo or to accompany chemo treatment?
6. Is it recommended that I have my ovaries removed for this type of breast cancer?
7. If it is suspected that I will have chemo, can I have a port installed during my surgery?
8. What type of anesthesia will be administered for the surgery?
9. Will I go home with a surgically inserted drain?
10. When will my first follow-up appointment be after the surgery?
11. Will I be required to have radiation treatment?
12. If it is deemed applicable when will chemo begin?
13. When should I be able to drive again?
14. Can you call in the prescription for pain medication the day before my surgery?
15. What type of pain or discomfort may happen after the surgery?
16. What side effects do you recommend I call the doctor for?
17. When will I be able to take a shower after the surgery?
18. What is cellulitis and what should I know about this as it relates to breast surgery?
19. What are the signals that I may be experiencing lymphedema and what should I do to minimize the risk of it occurring?
20. What is auxiliary cording and what are the symptoms?
21. Are there any preventative health maintenance appointments I should have before beginning treatment? Ex- dental work, etc.
22. What type of personal assistance will I need during/after treatment?
23. What are the types of reconstruction surgeries available to me and what are the risks associated with each?

QUESTIONS TO ASK THE ONCOLOGIST

1. Now that surgery is complete, what is the stage of my cancer and what is the official type of breast cancer that I have?

2. Is it recommended that I have any preventative surgeries to accompany my cancer treatment?

3. What maintenance appointments should I have before beginning chemo? (Ex dental, vaccinations) dental, vaccinations)

4. How many rounds of chemo will I have?

5. Which chemo medications are recommended, why is this drug recommended for me and what are the side effects of chemo medications? 6. Will I be required to have radiation treatment following chemo?

7. What can I do to reduce the side effects associated with metal mouth and mouth sores?

8. What can I do to reduce the symptoms of acid reflux? Both natural remedies as well as prescriptions?

9. What can I do to reduce the chances of UTIs?

10. How will we know if the chemo is working for my cancer?

11. What are some of the reasons we would stop chemotreatment?

12. Will I be on steroids or anti-nauseous medications days prior to chemo day and what is the regimen we will follow?

13. Can I bring a caregiver with me to my infusion appointments?

14. What type of physical changes should I expect to occur while on chemotherapy?

15. What type of mental changes may occur while on chemotherapy?

16. What is chemo brain fog and what are tips to improve mental clarity?

17. Will I be on medication to increase my white blood cells?

18. What impact can chemo have on my heart?

19. What can I do to prevent or minimize neuropathy?

QUESTIONS TO ASK THE RADIOLOGIST

1. How many rounds of radiation are required?
2. What type of pain or discomfort may occur during radiation treatment?
3. What can I do to protect my skin during treatment?
4. What are the risks associated with radiation treatment?
5. What are some of the long effects of radiation treatment?